Semen Analysis

A PRACTICAL GUIDE

Anne M. Jequier FRCS FRCOG

Senior Lecturer in Obstetrics and Gynaecology,
University of Nottingham

Joan P. Crich AIMLS

Senior Medical Laboratory Scientific Officer,
Department of Pathology,
City Hospital, Nottingham

BLACKWELL SCIENTIFIC PUBLICATIONS

OXFORD LONDON EDINBURGH

BOSTON PALO ALTO MELBOURNE

This book is dedicated to

Professor Roger Cotton

in gratitude for all his kindness, enthusiasm and help
over the past 10 years.

© 1986 by
Blackwell Scientific Publications
Editorial offices:
Osney Mead, Oxford, OX2 0EL
8 John Street, London, WC1N 2ES
23 Ainslie Place, Edinburgh, EH3 6AJ
52 Beacon Street, Boston
  Massachusetts 02108, USA
667 Lytton Avenue, Palo Alto
  California 94301, USA
107 Barry Street, Carlton
  Victoria 3053, Australia

First published 1986

Printed in Great Britain by The Alden
Press

DISTRIBUTORS

USA
  Blackwell Mosby Book Distributors
  11830 Westline Industrial Drive
  St Louis, Missouri 63141

Canada
  The C.V. Mosby Company
  5240 Finch Avenue East,
  Scarborough, Ontario

Australia
  Blackwell Scientific Publications
    (Australia) Pty Ltd
  107 Barry Street
  Carlton, Victoria 3053

British Library
Cataloguing in Publication Data

Jequier, Anne
  Semen analysis: a practical guide.
  1. Semen—Analysis—Laboratory
    manuals
  I. Title   II. Crich, Joan
  612'.61   QP255

ISBN 0-632-01591-8

Contents

Preface

Semen analysis is frequently the 'Cinderella' investigation of many pathology laboratories. It is often performed by staff who have little understanding of the physiology of seminal fluid itself and of the spermatozoa contained within it. As a consequence, inadequate, inappropriate or even erroneous information may be given to a clinician which can thus detrimentally influence his management of a couple's infertility.

With these problems in mind, it was decided that a book describing all the steps that can be taken to analyse semen could be of help to laboratories and may also be of assistance to the many clinicians involved in the management of infertility. We have tried to compile a simple handbook which not only describes the techniques used in the analysis of semen, but which also explains why such information is needed by the clinician and also outlines the underlying pathophysiological processes that may cause these abnormalities in semen quality. Included in this book are many of the less frequently used tests employed to establish the fertility of semen as these may, on occasions, be of help to those who are involved in semen analysis. There is also a chapter concerned with the cryopreservation of sperm and the organization of an AID bank.

The main object of this handbook is to provide practical help to those who are involved in the analysis of semen. However, we hope that it will also be of value to the clinicians who are involved in the treatment of the infertile couple.

1

The Anatomy of the Male Reproductive Tract

In order to understand the way semen is formed, it is important to have some idea of the anatomy of the male reproductive tract and in particular the structure of the accessory glands which are so important in the formation of semen.

Testes

Each testis is an ovoid organ normally measuring some 5 cm in length. Each testis lies in the scrotum on either side of a septum that divides the scrotal cavity into two halves.

The outer covering of each testis consists of a thick rigid fibrous capsule called the *tunica albuginea*. This thick capsule cannot distend and thus any disease or injury of the testis that produces oedema, can result in ischaemic damage to the spermatogenic elements within the testis (Fig. 1.1).

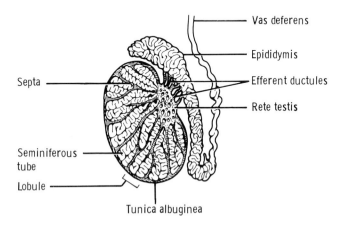

Fig. 1.1. The testis, its excurrent ducts together with the epididymal duct and the vas deferens.

1

Immediately beneath the tunica albuginea is a vascular layer
known as the *tunica vasculosa*. It is this layer that bleeds during any
operation on the testis in which the tunica albuginea is incised.

Arising from the tunica albuginea and extending into the substance of the testes are a series of fibrous septa which divide the testis
into lobules. Lying within the confines of these lobules are several
blind-ended or looped tubules. These are known as the *seminiferous
tubules* and it is inside their lumen that the development and production of spermatozoa takes place. Along the posterior border of the
testis, the tunica albuginea becomes thickened and indents the testis
to form the fibrous *mediastinum testis*. Within the mediastinum is a
complex system of channels which make up the *rete testis* (Fig. 1.2).

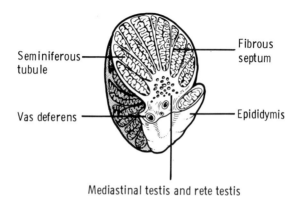

Mediastinal testis and rete testis

Fig. 1.2. A transverse section of testis showing the rete testis and its relationships
with the epididymis and the vas deferens.

Each testis contains between 200 and 300 seminiferous tubules.
Their total length when added together is estimated to be 70–80 cm
(*Gray's Anatomy*, 1973). Each tubule forms a loop within a lobule of the
testes and the two ends of this loop join together close to the mediastinum to form the straight (as opposed to the convoluted) seminiferous
tubule. These straight seminiferous tubules are also known as the
tubuli recti. Each seminiferous tubule now empties into the network of
channels that form the rete testis ('rete' means network), within the
mediastinum of the testis. Apart from forming channels that lead out
of the testis, the exact function of the rete is unknown. The presence of
myoid elements around the channels forming the rete testis may result
in the active expulsion of the sperm from the testis. There is good

evidence that disorders of the rete testis may result in male infertility (Guerin *et al.*, 1981).

Epididymis

The *epididymis* lies along the postero-lateral border of each testis. It is made up of tubules packed together in loose connective tissue. It consists of an upper portion known as the head (or caput), a middle portion known as the body (or corpus) and a lower portion known as the tail (or cauda) (Fig. 1.2).

Out of the upper pole of the testis emerge some 15–20 *efferent ductules* which act as the excurrent ducts of the testis. These ducts are very fine and are lined by a ciliated epithelium. They form part of the caput of the epididymis. Each efferent ductule empties into the upper end of a larger duct known as the *epididymal duct* which lies tightly coiled up alongside the testis and forms the body and most of the tail of the epididymis. The epididymal duct is very long (when uncoiled it may reach 6 m in length) and plays an extremely important role in the maturation of sperm. It is also lined by a ciliated epithelium which is both absorptive and secretory in function (Fig. 1.3).

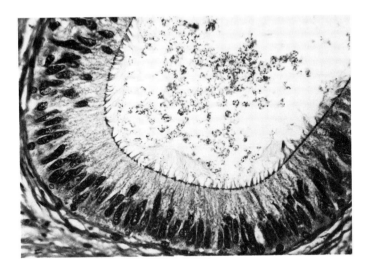

Fig. 1.3. A photomicrograph of the epididymal duct in the region of the caput of the epididymis. A highly ciliated epithelium is shown as well as cells that can undertake both secretory and absorptive activity. (Original magnification × 400.) With permission from Jequier, A. M. (1986) *Infertility in the Male*, p. 7. Churchill Livingstone, Edinburgh.

Within the tail of the epididymis, the epididymal duct increases its diameter but remains convoluted to form the *vas deferens*. After the vas deferens has emerged from the tail of the epididymis, it looses its convolutions and as a straight duct passes upwards out of the scrotum within the spermatic cord. The vas deferens is powerfully contractile and has a thick muscle coat (Fig. 1.4). Its epithelium is also ciliated but the ciliation is much less dense than that seen in the epididymal duct. It is this section of the vas deferens that is transected during a vasectomy.

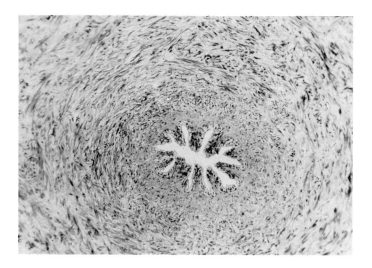

Fig. 1.4. A photomicrograph of a vas deferens showing the thick muscle wall and ciliated epithelium. (Original magnification × 100.)

Vas deferens and distal excurrent ducts

The vas deferens now passes up through the *inguinal canal* and into the pelvis. Behind the bladder, the vas dilates to form a chamber known as the *ampulla*. It is here, as well as in the vas deferens and in the cauda of the epididymis, that the sperm are stored.

Each ampulla then narrows and joins with the duct of the *seminal vesicle* (Fig. 1.5). Each seminal vesicle lies behind the bladder and is a sacculated pouch about 5 cm in length. Basically each vesicle consists of a tube coiled up on itself and which contains several blind-ended diverticula (Fig. 1.6). The seminal vesicles have a thick muscular coat which contracts powerfully at ejaculation. They are lined by a

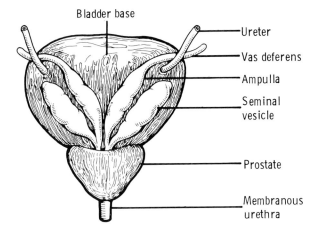

Fig. 1.5. The back of the bladder showing the relationship between the ureters, vasa deferentia and the seminal vesicles.

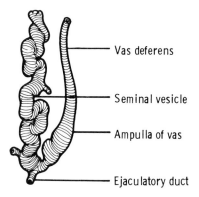

Fig. 1.6. A blind-ended seminal vesicle and its junction with the vas deferens on the same side to form an ejaculatory duct.

columnar epithelium containing goblet cells. Their secretions make up a large part of the seminal fluid.

The junction of the duct of the seminal vesicle with the ampulla of the vas deferens forms the *ejaculatory ducts*. These small ducts, which are only 2 cm in length, pass forwards and downwards between the median and lateral lobes of the prostate to open as slit-like orifices within the prostatic urethra. The raised portion of the urethra where these ducts open is known as the *verumontanum* (Fig. 1.7).

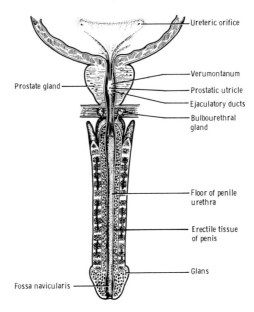

Ureteric orifice

Verumontanum

Prostate gland

Prostatic utricle

Ejaculatory ducts

Bulbourethral gland

Floor of penile urethra

Erectile tissue of penis

Glans

Fossa navicularis

Fig. 1.7. The urethra and some of the glands that make a contribution to the seminal fluid volume. The urethral glands open into the roof of the penile urethra and thus cannot be shown in this figure.

Prostate gland

The *prostate gland* is a glandular organ enclosed within a muscle coat which contracts at ejaculation. The prostate surrounds the posterior urethra and is divided into three lobes namely the median lobe and two lateral lobes. The secretions of the prostate which are expelled during ejaculation, enter the prostatic urethra by a series of small ducts which drain the main part of the gland and also the submucosal and mucosal areas of the prostate which surround the urethra (Fig. 1.8). Concretions or calculi are often seen within the acini of the prostate and these may occasionally be seen in semen. Like the seminal vesicles the prostate makes an important contribution to semen.

Bulbo-urethral glands

The *bulbo-urethral* glands are two small lobulated glands which secrete mostly mucus and which open into the membranous urethra (Fig. 1.7).

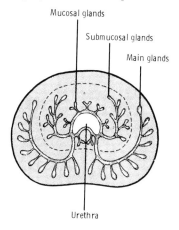

Mucosal glands

Submucosal glands

Main glands

Urethra

Fig. 1.8. The prostate gland and the mode of entry of its secretions into the prostatic urethra.

Urethral glands

The *urethral glands* are very small mucus-secreting glands that open into the roof of the penile urethra and are particularly numerous in a dilatation of the urethra that occurs at the end of the urethra known as the fossa navicularis.

This brief review of the anatomy of the male genital tract has been included as it is felt that an understanding of the abnormalities of semen can only be complete if it is put into the context of disordered morphology as well as disordered function. For this reason, spermatogenesis and the morphology of the sperm will be outlined in Chapters 2 and 3.

References

Gray's Anatomy (1973) The Testes. p. 1338. 35th Edition. Johnston, T. B. & Whillis, J. (eds). Longmans, Green and Co.

Guerin, J-F., Czyba, J-C., Perrin, P. & Rollet, J. (1981) Les obstruction congenitales ou aquises de l'epididyme humain: Etude de la mobilite des spermatozoides en amont de l'obstruction. *Bulletin de l'Association des Anatomistes.* **65**, 297–306.

2

Testicular Function
and Spermatogenesis

The testis, like the ovary, has two main functions: it produces hormones, in particular testosterone, and it produces gametes in the form of spermatozoa.

Most of the volume of the testis is made up of the looped or blind-ended seminiferous tubules which lie packed in connective tissue within the confines of the fibrous septa that form the lobules of the testis. Lying singly but more often in groups within the connective tissue that binds the convolutions of the tubules together, are the Leydig cells (otherwise known as interstitial cells). The Leydig cells are the prime source of the male sex hormone, testosterone. The seminiferous tubules are the site of sperm production.

Leydig cells

The Leydig cells are irregularly shaped cells with rather granular cytoplasm. There appear to be two main populations of Leydig cells some of which secrete far more testosterone than others (Payne *et al.*, 1980). The pituitary hormone, luteinising hormone, perhaps more familiarly known as LH, acts on the Leydig cells to stimulate the production of testosterone. This androgen is released into the circulation and acts as a negative 'feedback' on the pituitary to suppress or modulate further LH secretion (Fig. 2.1). Very high concentrations of testosterone are therefore found close to the basement membrane of the seminiferous tubule: indeed the intra-testicular concentration of testosterone is many times higher than the concentration of testosterone in blood. Thus the pharmacological administration of testosterone can in no way replace or mimic the function of the Leydig cells.

Seminiferous tubule

The convolutions of the seminiferous tubules lie closed together within

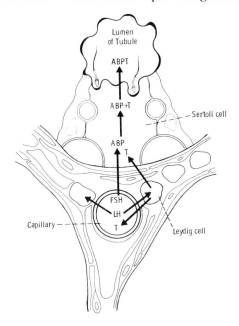

Fig 2.1. A diagrammatic representation of the action of the two pituitary gonadotrophins on the testis.

the lobules of the testis and are held in loose connective tissue. They are separated by blood vessels, lymphatics, nerves and by the Leydig cells themselves. The wall of each tubule is made up of myoid cells of limited contractility and also of fibrous tissue.

The basic unit that lines the seminiferous tubule is the *Sertoli cell*. These tall, irregularly shaped cells with large nuclei that contain prominent nucleoli act as a support to spermatogenesis but are also a source of hormone. The Sertoli cells extend from the basement membrane of the tubule to the lumen. Between them lie the developing gametes in various stages of development. One interesting feature of the Sertoli cells is that each cell is joined to its neighbour by 'tight junctions' which prevent any passage of substances between their cell walls. Thus any substance must pass through the Sertoli cell before it can reach the lumen of the seminiferous tubule.

The Sertoli cell is sensitive to stimulation by the other pituitary hormone follicle stimulating hormone (FSH). In response to the action of FSH, the Sertoli cells manufacture a protein called androgen binding protein (ABP) which has a high affinity for testosterone (Hansson *et al.*, 1974). The testosterone produced by the Leydig cells passes through the basement of the seminiferous tubule and into the Sertoli cells where it binds to the *androgen binding protein*. Interestingly, some of the testosterone is also converted, within the Sertoli cell, to oestrogen (Dorrington *et al.*, 1978). The testosterone bound to androgen binding protein is secreted by the Sertoli cell into the lumen of the tubule, from where the testosterone–androgen binding protein complex is transported out of the testis and into the efferent ductules and the epididymal duct (Hansson *et al.*, 1974). This mechanism thus provides the excurrent ducts of the testis with the high concentrations of testosterone that are needed for their normal function. It is also believed that the action of FSH on the Sertoli cell may stimulate the production of a hormone or group of hormones called *inhibin* (Franchimont *et al.*, 1975). The main action of inhibin is to provide a negative feedback mechanism which will reduce, and therefore control, the pituitary secretion of FSH (Steinberger & Steinberger, 1976).

Contained within the Sertoli cell are quantities of a substance called *tubulin* that acts as a cytoskeleton and which may help to support the Sertoli cell and germinal elements lying alongside it. Sertoli cells also contain large amounts of rough endoplasmic reticulum whose function is protein synthesis. A complex Golgi apparatus is also present. It is therefore clear that the Sertoli cell plays a very active role within the seminiferous tubule and does not merely provide passive support for the developing spermatozoa.

Spermatogenesis

Cells known as *spermatogonia* form the basic stem cell from which spermatozoa develop. Before it can become a sperm, each spermatogonium must undergo radical morphological changes and meiotic division. The spermatogonia lie between the Sertoli cells in contact with the basement membrane of the seminiferous tubule. During the course of their development, all the germinal elements lie in close contact with the Sertoli cells: indeed considerable invagination of the Sertoli cells is produced by the developing sperm (Fig. 2.2).

The spermatogonia first undergo mitotic division in order to increase their numbers and enter the spematogenic process. Four types of spermatogonia may be seen in the human testis: long, pale and dark type A spermatogonia, and type B spermatogonia. It is likely that all four types of spermatogonia are capable of undergoing division to become *primary spermatocytes*.

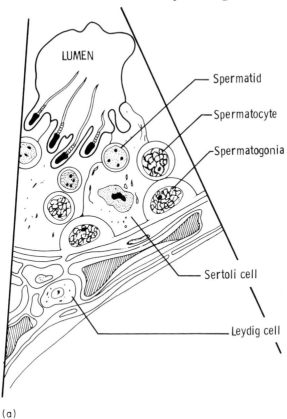

(a)

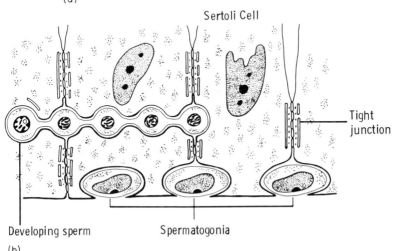

(b)

Fig. 2.2. (a) Developing gametes. (b) Their relationship to the 'tight junctions' between the Sertoli cells. With kind permission from Huckins *c.* (1975). In *Infertility in the Male*, p. 110, Lipshultz, L. I. & Howards, S. S. (eds). Churchill Livingstone, Edinburgh.

The *primary spermatocytes* now undergo differentiation during the course of meiotic division to become *secondary spermatocytes*. The division of the secondary spermatocytes to form spermatids completes reduction division. The spermatids thus have a haploid chromosome content. The process of differentiation of a spermatogonium into a spermatid is known as spermatogenesis.

Spermiogenesis

The morphological changes that take place during the differentiation of the spermatid into the spermatozoon is a process called *spermiogenesis* and must be differentiated from spermatogenesis. During spermiogenesis, the nucleus of the spermatid becomes eccentric and the chromatin condenses. The cell elongates and the axial filament forms. The cytoplasm around the axial filament reduces in amount and finally disappears. Finally the mitochondria become applied to the proximal portion of the tail and a mature spermatid is formed (Fig. 2.3).

Spermiation

The process whereby a mature spermatid frees itself from the Sertoli cell and thus enters the lumen of the tubule as a spermatozoon is known as *spermiation*. It almost certainly involves the active participation of the Sertoli cell. It may also involve actual cell movement and for this the tubulin cytoskeleton within the Sertoli cell may be of importance. During the process of spermiation, portions of the cytoplasm of the Sertoli cell may remain as part of the spermatozoon (a morphological feature present on immature sperm in semen) known as a cytoplasmic droplet.

Speed of Sperm Maturation

This varies between different species but appears to be relatively constant in man. The time taken for the differentiation of a spermatogonium into a mature spermatid is estimated to be 70 ± 4 days (Heller & Clermont, 1964). The process of spermiation and the journey of a sperm through the excurrent ducts of the testis to a site where it can be included in an ejaculate, is thought to take a further 10–14 days.

The production of spermatozoa is a complex process. However, a basic understanding of the process of sperm production is necessary in

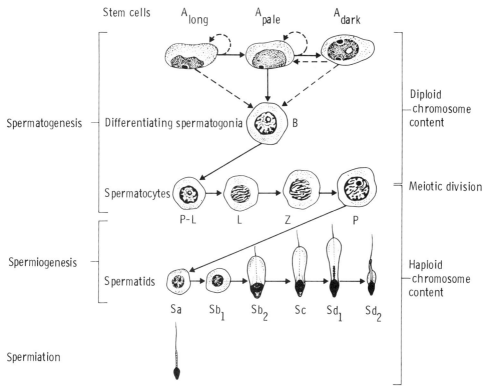

Fig. 2.3. A diagrammatic representation of the process of spermatogenesis, spermiogenesis and spermiation during which the developing germ cells undergo mitotic and then meiotic division to halve their chromosome content. With kind permission from Huckins C. (1975). In *Infertility in the Male,* p. 108, Lipshultz, L. I. & Howards, S. S. (eds). Churchill Livingstone, Edinburgh.

order to recognize many of the immature germinal elements that can occasionally be seen in semen and also to understand that, being a lengthy process, quantitative changes in sperm production may take some time to become apparent in a sample of semen.

References

Dorrington, J. H., Fritz, I. B. & Armstrong, D. T. (1978) Steroidogenesis by Granulosa and Sertoli Cells. *International Journal of Andrology* **1** (Suppl 2), 53–64.

Franchimont, P., Chari, S., Hagelstein, M-T. & Duraiswami, S. (1975) Existence of a Follicle Stimulating Hormone inhibitory factor 'Inhibin' in bull seminal plasma. *Nature* **257**, 402–4.

Hansson, V., Trygstad, O., French, F. S., Tindall, D. J., Weddington, S., Petrusz, P., Nayfeh, S. N. & Ritzen, E. M. (1974) Androgen transport and receptor mechanisms in testis and epididymis. *Nature* **250**, 387–91.

Heller, C. G., & Clermont, Y. (1964) Kinetics of the germinal epithelium in man. *Recent Progress in Hormonal Research* **20**, 545–75.

Payne, A. H., Downing, J. R. & Wong, K-L. (1980) Luteinising Hormone receptors and testosterone synthesis in two distinct populations of Leydig cells. *Endocrinology* **106**, 1424–9.

Steinberger, A. & Steinberger, E. (1976) Secretion of an FSH-inhibiting factor by cultured Sertoli cells. *Endocrinology* **99**, 918–21.

3

Morphology of Human Spermatozoa

In order to achieve fertilization, for which it must enter, and journey a considerable distance through the female genital tract, the sperm must not only be motile but also be capable of forward progression. The sperm must therefore be a very complex cell. Spermatozoa are also very small and much of their morphology cannot be determined without the use of the electron microscope. The following description of the structure of a human sperm makes use, to a large part, of the higher resolution offered by electron microscopy (Fawcett, 1975).

Sperm head

Each normal human spermatozoon is made up of two main parts, a head and a tail (Fig. 3.1). The sperm *head* is flat and measures approximately 4.5 μm in length, 3 μm in width and 1.5 μm thick. The sperm head is therefore about half the size of a red blood cell. The head consists of two main parts, the nucleus and the acrosome. The darkly staining nucleus holds the whole of the chromatin content of the sperm and virtually fills the whole head. The anterior two-thirds of the head is enveloped by two membranes known as the inner and the outer acrosomal membranes between which lies the *acrosome* itself. The acrosome is made up of a collection of many enzymes that will aid penetration of the zona pellucida by the sperm. Breakdown of the outer acrosomal membrane and release of these enzymes occurs, in the human, in the female genital tract. This phenomenon is known as the *acrosome reaction* and is one of the activities which make up a process known as *capacitation*. The posterior one-third of the sperm head is often known as the post acrosomal region and is separated from the anterior two-thirds (or acrosome region) by a furrow. This posterior part of the nucleus is covered by the double layered post acrosomal lamina.

The *connecting piece* is a small area in a very short segment that joins the head to the tail. This region of the sperm is important as it

15

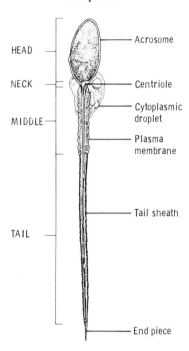

HEAD

NECK

MIDDLE

TAIL

Acrosome

Centriole

Cytoplasmic
droplet

Plasma
membrane

Tail sheath

End piece

Fig. 3.1. The structure of a human spermatozoon.

contains the proximal centriole which, if malformed, will render a sperm immotile and thus be a cause of infertility. The *proximal centriole* is only visible on electron microscopy.

Sperm tail

The *tail* of the sperm consists of three parts: the midpiece, the principle piece and the terminal segment. Overall the tail measures around 50 μm. The tail, of course, is the means by which the sperm moves. The whole length of the tail contains a central contractile unit known as the *axoneme* (Fig. 3.2). The axoneme is made up of nine doublet microtubules which surround two single microtubules giving the well-known '9+2' configuration. This arrangement continues throughout the length of the tail to the terminal segment. Each microtubule is made up of units of the contractile substance tubulin.

The outer doublets of tubulin consist of two subunits, A and B. Subunit A is a complete microtubule while subunit B is incomplete and has its ends joined to subunit A. Each subunit A is joined to 'arms'

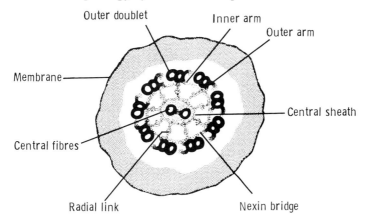

Fig. 3.2. The central axoneme of a spermatozoon. This pattern is common to all cilia. Abnormalities of this configuration of tubulin may be a cause of sperm immotility and infertility.

made up of *dynein* which is a substance that can convert chemical energy into contractility. Each of these arms reach out to subunit B of the next outer doublet. Abnormalities or absence of the dyenin arms are a common cause of poor sperm movement and consequent infertility. Also arising from subunit A are *nexin links* that connect with adjacent doublets. The central single tubules are surrounded by a central sheath. A radial link or spoke joins each outer doublet with the central sheath. The normal arrangement and morphology of these microtubules and their interconnections are vital for normal movement of sperm and therefore for normal fertility. The axoneme is only visible using transmission electron microscopy.

In the *middle piece*, this central axoneme is surrounded by a closely packed helix of mitochondria which are contained within a fibrous sheath. The close relationship of the mitochondria with the tubule system allows for the easy transfer of energy.

The *principle piece* forms, at least in terms of length, the most important part of the tail. Indeed, it makes up more than 90% of the length of the tail. In the principle piece, the mitochondrial covering is lost but the fibrous sheath continues to cover the tail giving it a ribbed appearance.

At the terminal segment, the fibrous sheath disappears leaving the axonemal tubules covered only by a plasma membrane.

Due to its complexity, abnormalities of the sperm tail are frequent and can often be a cause of poor sperm movement and therefore of reproductive failure. Electron microscopy has an important part to play in the diagnosis of male infertility especially in relation to disorders of sperm movement (Zamboni *et al.*, 1971) but it must be remembered that electron microscopy of sperm is both time-consuming and expensive. Where morphological assessment by electron microscopy is indicated in semen analysis and where the description of morphological abnormalities of sperm by light microscopy will suffice, is discussed in a later section. There is however an important role for electron microscopy in the examination of sperm and for this reason, a knowledge of the anatomy of the sperm is important.

References

Fawcett, D. W. (1975) The Mammalian Spermatozoa. *Developmental Biology* **44**, 394–436.

Zamboni, L., Zemjanis, R. & Stefani, M. (1971) The fine structure of monkey and human spermatozoa. *Anatomical Record* **169**, 129–53.

4

Secretions that make up Semen

Semen is a grey opalescent fluid which is formed at ejaculation. It consists of a suspension of spermatozoa in seminal plasma. Although semen contains spermatozoa it is not solely testicular in origin. In fact, semen is made up of the secretions of all the accessory glands of the male genital tract as well as a testicular component. The other secretions that go to make up semen are produced by the seminal vesicles, the prostate and also the bulbo-urethral and urethral glands. Even the duct systems contribute in a minor way to the volume of the ejaculate, and the epididymal duct adds biochemical substances to semen which are important for the normal function of the sperm. The testicular contribution, volumetrically, forms a relatively small proportion of the ejaculate (Table 4.1). It is clear that either quantitative or qualitative changes in one or more of these secretions that form semen, may have profound effects not only on the concentration of sperm in the ejaculate but also on sperm function. Thus, as will be seen later, reproductive failure may be the result of a pathology of one of the accessory glands rather than any abnormality of sperm production.

Table 4.1. The percentage contribution of each of the secretions that make up the seminal fluid (from Lundquist, 1949)

Source of secretion	% Ejaculate
Testes	5
Seminal Vesicles	46–80
Prostate	13–33
Bulbo-urethral and urethral gland	2–5

Each of the contributions that make up semen come together when, during intercourse, they are individually propelled into the posterior

urethra in a process known as *emission*. These secretions do not mix
however, until they are expelled into the vagina from the urethra at
ejaculation, which quickly follows emission. However, during ejaculation each of the components that make up semen may be discharged
from the urethra in a predetermined sequence. Thus by carefully collecting semen as it is discharged, it is possible, at least in part, to
separate out the secretions that make up an ejaculate. Semen collected
in this way is known as *split ejaculate* (Eliasson, 1959). This type of
ejaculate provides useful information for the diagnosis of some causes
of infertility in the male.

It is now of value to consider each of the components of seminal
fluid and their sites of origin in more detail.

Testicular component of semen

The testicular component of semen is very important to fertility as, of
course, it contains the spermatozoa. However, in terms of volume it
only makes up around 5% or 0.2 ml of the final volume of the ejaculate
(Lundquist, 1949). Thus no significant reduction in volume is noticed
after vasectomy. In their passage through the seminiferous tubules
and the rete of the testis, the sperm are accompanied by a large variety
of chemical substances and some of these are not only important functionally but can be of value diagnostically.

Rete testis fluid, that is, the fluid arriving at the excurrent ducts of
the testis, is rich in adrogens. Testosterone which has been produced
by the Leydig cells under the influence of luteinising hormone (LH)
passes through the seminiferous tubular basement membrane and into
the Sertoli cells. There the testosterone binds to androgen binding
protein (ABP) which is manufactured within the Sertoli cells under the
influence of the other pituitary hormone, Follicle Stimulating
Hormone (FSH). The testosterone, bound to ABP is released into the
lumen of the seminiferous tubule and accompanies the spermatozoa
out of the testis (Hansson *et al.*, 1974). Another protein, namely transferrin, is also produced by the Sertoli cells and is found in rete testis
fluid. Its function in semen is not clear. A third important substance
present in rete testis fluid is also produced by the Sertoli cells and is
the hormone, or group of hormones, known as inhibin (Franchimont *et
al.*, 1975). This substance or perhaps group of substances, suppresses
the pituitary production of FSH and thus acts as an important feedback mechanism of FSH. Inhibin is very difficult to measure but its

assay is already being used in special centres for the diagnosis of disorders of fertility in men which are associated with dysfunction of the Sertoli cells.

The efferent ductules and the epididymal duct and their contribution to the semen

These duct systems add little to the semen in terms of volume. Indeed the efferent ductules remove water from the rete testis fluid and thus concentrate the spermatozoa. However, the epididymal duct adds many biochemical substances to the semen which are of great importance functionally to the spermatozoa (Turner, 1979). The best known of these substances is carnitine which is an important energy source for sperm (Cassilas, 1973). Carnitine is not manufactured by the epididymis but is concentrated by it (Brooks *et al.*, 1974). The conversion of carnitine to acetyl-carnitine acts as an important means of inducing motility in sperm. Inositol, which is a sugar, is also secreted into the epididymal duct (Voglemayr, 1974) but its function remains unclear. Inositol is however converted in the epididymal duct into phosphatidyl-inositol. Lipids and phospholipids are also present in high concentration in epididymal fluid and are there converted into glycerophosphocholine. There is also some evidence, at least in the rat, that the epididymal wall may be a site of the further androgen production (Hamilton, 1972).

The main feature of the spermatozoa as they pass down the epididymal duct is that they acquire some degree of motility. Indeed there is a substance called *epididymal motility protein* found in the bovine epididymal duct which coats the sperm and appears to induce motility (Brandt *et al.*, 1978).

Spermatozoa therefore undergo important changes in the epididymis. Epididymal pathology may thus cause major changes in the character and function of the spermatozoa in an ejaculate. One of the major changes that occur to spermatozoa in their passage down the epididymal duct is that they acquire an ability to fertilize oocytes, and it has been demonstrated in many experimental animals that sperm taken from the head of the epididymis cannot penetrate eggs while those taken from the tail of the epididymis fertilize eggs with ease (Bedford, 1966). These changes in the fertility potential of sperm relate closely to their motility (Hinton *et al.*, 1979).

Seminal vesicles and their secretions

In terms of volume, the secretions of the seminal vesicles are the most important contributions to the ejaculate.

The seminal vesicles are glands which lie at the back of the bladder and their ducts join with the vasa to form the ejaculatory duct. Their secretions make up between 40 and 80% of the ejaculatory volume (Lundquist, 1949). Aside from their volume, the secretions of the seminal vesicles contain biochemical substances which are important both functionally and diagnostically.

The best known substance secreted by the seminal vesicles is the sugar *fructose* (Mann, 1974). This is an important energy source for sperm and exclusion of the seminal vesicular component from the ejaculate will result in almost completely immotile sperm. Likewise, disorders of the seminal vesicles and a subsequent reduction in the fructose concentration in semen will also result in a reduced motility of the sperm (Eliasson, 1971). The seminal vesicles are also the main site of *prostaglandin* synthesis (Eliasson & Lindholmer, 1971) and this substance may also play a role in controlling sperm movement and sperm penetration of cervical mucus. The seminal vesicles also appear to be the source of the fibrinogen-like substance which is acted upon by the enzyme *vesiculase* to induce the clotting that occurs in semen (Gotterer *et al.*, 1955).

Prostatic contribution

The prostate secretes its contribution to semen straight into the urethra by means of multiple ducts that lie on and around the verumontanum in the prostatic urethra. The prostate contributes the second largest volume of fluid to the semen (Lundquist, 1949). The prostatic secretions are biochemically very active. They contain large numbers of enzymes which are involved with semen clotting and liquefaction (Gotterer *et al.*, 1955). These enzymes include vesiculase that induces clotting of semen and also the proteases which liquify semen. The subject of liquefaction of semen will be dealt with in more detail in a later chapter. Prostatic secretions also contain the bacteriostatic amine *spermine* which can form spermine phosphate whose crystals may be seen on microscopy of semen (Tabor & Tabor, 1964). Prostatic fluid also contains large amounts of *acid phosphatase*. This enzyme is very stable, and for this reason, is commonly used in forensic medicine as a marker of the presence of semen stains on clothes. Likewise citrates are abundant in prostatic secretions (Mann, 1964). It is also the prostate that is the source of high concentrations of both calcium and, in particular, zinc (Eliasson & Lindholmer, 1971).

Secretions of the bulbo-urethral and urethral glands

These glands open into the urethra more proximally and the volume of their combined secretions is small. The fluid secreted is rich in muco-proteins and the role of these glands may be solely to lubricate the urethra. However, although the contribution to semen is of little significance in the normal patient, it has been suggested that these secretions can occasionally contain specific antisperm antibodies. These glands may therefore indeed be of importance in the infertile patient. However, the whole problem of immune infertility and its detection in semen and serum will be discussed later in this book.

Seminal fluid is thus made up not only of spermatozoa but also of a wide range of different chemical substances (Table 4.2). It should

Table 4.2. Important biochemical substances that are present in each of the contributions to the ejaculate

Source	Important biochemical substances
Testes	Testosterone Androgen binding protein Transferrin Inhibin
Epdidymal ducts	Carnitine Inositol Lipids, glycerophosphorylcholine Epdidiymal motility protein
Seminal vesicles	Fructose Prostaglandins Substrate for the clotting of semen
Prostate	Proteases Spermine Acid phosphatase Citrate Calcium, zinc Vesiculase
Bulbo urethral and urethral glands	Mucoproteins, IgA

therefore be clear that any change in one of the secretions that go to
make up semen may produce major changes in the appearance of
semen as a whole. Such changes may alter profoundly not only the
physicochemical properties of the seminal fluid but also the activity
and thus the potential for fertilization of the spermatozoa. In performing a semen analysis, the differing role that each of these secretions,
individually or serially, may play in producing an abnormality of
semen must constantly be remembered. As will be seen later, such a
thought process when used in conjunction with semen analysis, may be
extremely helpful diagnostically. As diagnosis is the single most important factor in determining the correct management of an infertile
patient, the laboratory will therefore play a very important role in the
successful management of an infertile couple.

References

Bedford, J. M. (1966) Development of the fertilising ability of spermatozoa in the
    epididymis of the rabbit. *Experimental Zoology* **163**, 319–25.
Brandt, H., Acott, T. S., Johnson, D. J. & Hoskins, D. D. (1978) Evidence for an
    epididymal origin of bovine sperm forward motility protein. *Biological Reproduction*
    19, 830–5.
Brooks, D. E., Hamilton, D. W. & Malleck, A. H. (1974) Carnitine and glycerylphos-
    phorylcholine in the reproductive tract of the male rat. *Journal of Reproduction and
    Fertility* **36**, 141–60.
Cassilas, E. R. (1973) Accumulation of carnitine by bovine spermatozoa during matura-
    tion in the epididymis. *Journal of Biological Chemistry* **248**, 8227–33.
Eliasson, R. (1959) Studies on prostaglandin. Occurrence and formation and biological
    action. *Acta Physiologica Scandinavica* **46** (Suppl. 158), 1–73.
Eliasson, R. (1971) Standards for the investigation of human semen. *Andrologie* **3**, 49–
    64.
Eliasson, R. & Lindholmer, C. (1971) Zinc in human seminal plasma. *Andrologie* **3**, 147–
    53.
Franchimont, P., Chari, S., Hagelstein, M-T. & Duraiswami, S. (1975) Existence of a
    Follicle Stimulating Hormone inhibitory factor Inhibin in bull seminal plasma.
    Nature **257**, 402–4.
Gotterer, G., Ginsberg, D., Shulman, T., Banks, J. & Williams-Ashman, H. G. (1955)
    Enzymatic coagulation of semen. *Nature* **176**, 1209–11.
Hamilton, D. W. (1972) The mammalian epididymis. In Balin, H. & Glasser, S. (eds)
    Reproductive Biology, pp. 268–337. Excerpta Medica Amsterdam.
Hansson, V., Trygstad, O., French, F. S., McLean, W. S., Smith, A. A., Tindall, D. J.,
    Weddington, S. C., Petrusz, P., Nayfeh, S. N. & Ritzen, E. M. (1974) Androgen trans-
    port and receptor mechanisms in testis and epididymis. *Nature* **250**, 387–91.
Hinton, B. T., Dott, H. M. & Setchell, B. P. (1979) Measurement of the motility of rat
    spermatozoa collected by micropuncture from the testis and from different regions
    along the epididymis. *Journal of Reproduction and Fertility* **55**, 167–72.
Lundquist, F. (1949) Aspects of the biochemistry of human semen. *Acta Physiologica
    Scandinavica* **19** (Suppl. 66), 7–105.

Mann, T. (1974) Secretory function of the prostate, seminal vesicle and other male accessory organs of reproduction. *Journal of Reproduction and Fertility* **37**, 179–88.

Tabor, H. & Tabor, C. W. (1964) Spermidine, spermine and related amines. *Pharmacological Review* **16**, 245–300.

Turner, T. T. (1979) On the epididymis and its function. *Investigative Urology* **16**, 311–21.

Voglemayr, J. K. (1974) Alpha-chlorhydrin-induced changes in the distribution of free myo-inositol and prostaglandin F_2 and synthesis of phosphatidyl-inositol in the rat epididymis. *Biology of Reproduction* **2**, 593–600.

5

Sample Production for the Laboratory

Although infertility and its evaluation is probably the most common reason for a semen analysis, there are in fact many other indications for this procedure. Semen analysis, for example, is required in the routine follow up of patients who have undergone vasectomy and in such men, the semen will be repeatedly analysed until azoospermia has been confirmed. Semen needed for artificial insemination by husband (AIH) and artificial insemination by donor (AID) will also need examination as it is useless to inseminate or to store semen that has no potential for fertility. The storage of a husband's semen may be necessary if he is away from home for any length of time especially when the wife is undergoing complicated infertility therapy which would otherwise have to be postponed. Men whose future fertility is threatened, for example by the need for radiotherapy or chemotherapy in the treatment of cancer, may also wish to have their semen analysed with a view to its storage for future insemination.

Whatever the reason for the semen analysis, it is important to remember that the production of a specimen of semen for analysis may be, at least for some patients, distasteful, difficult and embarrassing. If these emotions are superimposed on the problems of infertility which inevitably may be associated with some feelings of inadequacy, it is clear that to such patients, the production of a semen specimen may be a very stressful and unpleasant event. For this reason, it is very important to relax the patient and allow the production of the specimen to take place in surroundings which are the most comfortable both emotionally and physically for the patient. The production of semen for analysis in a situation of stress can lead to inadequate ejaculation. This may well result in the production of an incomplete specimen which will in turn cause misdiagnosis as to the evaluation of a couple's infertility. Also, unhappy events such as this may well lead to poor compliance and attendance at the Infertility Clinic. As a result, both the diagnosis and treatment of the couple's infertility will be

26

unsatisfactory. For all these reasons, the collection of semen specimens must be organized by experienced staff.

Length of abstinence

The length of abstinence prior to the production of a semen specimen alters, to some extent, both the sperm numbers and their motility but for this to happen the length of abstinence must be either very short or very long (Eliasson, 1965; Mortimer *et al.*, 1982). However, provided that the specimen is not produced within 24 hours of a previous ejaculation, and the length of abstinence is known, 2–3 days is a quite adequate length of abstinence for the proper assessment of semen quality. One could argue that the length of abstinence should equal that which occurs normally for the patient: if sexual intercourse normally occurs 2 or 3 times per week, then 2–3 days abstinence ought to reflect the semen quality produced during normal married life.

Site of production of the semen specimen

There is no doubt that it is much simpler for the laboratory staff if a patient produces a specimen of semen in the hospital. The specimen can then be brought straight to the bench for examination. However, semen analyses are not being performed for the benefit of the laboratory staff; they are being performed for the benefit of the patient. As has already been pointed out, stress may be a problem to many men in the production of a semen specimen. For this reason, the patient must be allowed, within reason, to choose where he wishes to produce the specimen. If he prefers to produce the specimen at home, so be it. If, however, he lives a long way away and is happy to produce the specimen in hospital, then a room should be provided which is quiet, secluded and which will guarantee total privacy.

Time of production of semen specimen

A semen specimen is best produced in the morning for, as will be seen later, an assessment of motility 6 hours after production is of value. However, if this proves difficult for the patient for any reason, then a specimen produced in the afternoon will have to suffice. Indeed, what may be gained in information by pressurising a patient to produce a specimen in the morning, can be lost in misinformation occurring as a result of the production of an incomplete specimen. Especially today, journeys to the hospital may jeopardize future employment or at least induce a fear of job loss. Pressure on the patient in this manner may also make the patient untruthful about the time of production of a specimen. For the same reason, there should never be an appointment system for seminal analyses: the presence of any 'deadline' for semen production is best avoided.

Method of production of a semen specimen

There is no doubt that the production of semen by masturbation usually results in a specimen that is complete and otherwise uncontaminated. However, there are a few patients who find masturbation difficult or offensive and others who have religious objections to it. For these patients, the semen must be collected in different ways.

Such patients may elect to produce such specimens by coitus interruptus. This method, otherwise known as the 'withdrawal' method can be used. However, in order to get the specimen to the laboratory, intercourse has to take place in laboratory hours and this may be inconvenient to the patient. More important, collection of the specimen may be mistimed and part of the ejaculate may thus be lost. Ordinary condoms must *never* be used to collect semen specimens. Most condoms contain spermicidal powder which swiftly obliterates all sperm motility. Many of these powders have characteristically shaped crystals and can be identified during microscopy of the semen. Even plain rubber condoms damage sperm motility due to the presence of toxic hydrocarbons that exist between the interslices of the rubber. Silastic condoms, however, are available and do not harm sperm but are difficult to obtain. It should be remembered that even if non-toxic condoms are used, part of the specimen can easily be lost on its transfer from the condom to the container. Another way of obtaining a semen specimen from coitus is by the use of a home-made condom made from ordinary kitchen 'plastic film' (Jequier, unpublished). This kitchen film seems to be completely non-toxic to sperm and provided they are transferred fairly quickly into their container and given access to air, very good semen specimens can be obtained.

Containers used for the semen specimen

All patients should be provided with containers for their semen samples. Jars obtained at home by the patients have usually been washed out with detergents which are highly toxic to sperm. Moreover, such containers may also be wet and water is equally lethal to sperm. Of course, it must be emphasized that the container should be correctly labelled.

The semen sample containers should be wide necked: it is difficult for a patient to ejaculate into a narrow necked container (Fig. 5.1). Above all, the container must be *clean*. The jar can be made of plastic or glass. It is important to remember that there must not be a rubber lining to the lid as contact between the rubber lid and the sperm may result in sperm death.

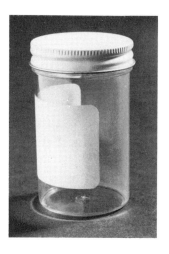

Fig. 5.1. The plastic pot, with a diameter of at least 7 cm, recommended for the collection of a semen specimen. The metal top must *not* contain a rubber liner. (With permission from Jequier, A. M. (1986) *Infertility in the Male*, p. 23. Churchill Livingstone, Edinburgh.)

Transport of the specimen to the hospital

Sperm are easily damaged by either excessive heat or excessive cold. Although excessive heat is unusual in this country, semen specimens should not be left for any length of time in direct sunlight. Similarly, in winter, a handbag or an outside pocket can be at too low a temperature for sperm survival.

The semen specimen therefore should be brought to the laboratory at close to body temperature and the best place to transport it is in an inside jacket or waistcoat pocket.

The card that should accompany the specimen of semen

Many people have devised quite complex cards for use with semen specimens. Probably all that is really needed, apart from the patient's name and an indication of where the report should be sent, is the date and time of production of the specimen and the date of the last ejaculation or sexual intercourse. It is, of course, also useful to know how the specimen was produced, that is, by masturbation or coitus interruptus.

Delivery to the laboratory

It is best, but not essential that the semen specimen is delivered to the laboratory within 2 hours of production. However, on its arrival at the laboratory reception area, a specimen whose temperature has previously been well maintained may now inadvertently be allowed to cool. The time spent by semen specimens in a cold corridor of a pathology department is often enough to produce quite profound artifactual changes in sperm motility. Thus rapid transfer of the semen to the department concerned with its analysis after its arrival at the laboratory is important.

Artifacts that can occur in the production of a semen sample

There are a number of abnormalities that can occur in semen which are due simply to errors or faults in the collection of semen.

'Missed the jar'

Such specimens can often be recognized by the associated reduction in volume, although as will be seen later, there are many other real causes of low-volume ejaculate. The qualitative changes in the semen associated with this problem will depend on what part of the specimen 'missed the jar' (Fig. 5.2). Loss of semen can also occur when the jar is accidently upset or dropped.

OBS & GYNAE (B Floor) UNIVERSITY HOSPITAL NOTTM		Use Block Letters or affix label
Specimen *Semen sample*	Report to be sent to:–	Hosp. No.: .... Surname: .... First Names: ....
Date of last ejaculation		DOB/Age: ....
Time of production		....

Volume *0·4* ml	pH *6·8*	Liquefaction		
Count *4·3x10⁶*/ml		Total sperm count	Clumping	
	% Motility	Motile sperm count	Progressive Activity	
3 hours	*10%*		*Poor*	
6 hours	*0%*			
% Abnormal forms *70%*			Types of Abnormal forms	
Invasion Tests				
			M.A.R. Test	
Additional Information			Signature .... Date	~P 108~
			FERTILITY ANALYSIS	

Fig. 5.2. A typical analysis from semen where most of the specimen had 'missed the jar'. Note the reduced volume, low pH and poor motility. Without knowledge of the presence of this artifact, this patient could have been thought to be infertile.

In such cases, the secretions which make up the ejaculate will be mixed as the only sign of this accident will be a reduced volume of ejaculate. Occasionally a patient will try to retrieve a specimen from the floor and this may be revealed by finding a whole variety of particular matter in the specimen!

Condom collection

Unless previously warned, many patients will collect their semen specimens during intercourse in a condom. Such specimens will show almost no sperm motility and if the condom has been coated with a spermacidal powder, crystals of these agents may be seen in the seminal fluid. Such crystals should not however be confused with the crystals of talcum powder which may also be seen in semen but which appear to do little harm to spermatozoa.

Temperature extremes

Apart from a reduction in motility and cell death, extremes of temperature have no other apparent morphological effect on spermatozoa.

Contamination of the jar containing the semen specimen

The most usual contaminant of the jar in which the specimen is collected is water and this will rapidly kill sperm. However as has already been stated, soap, detergents and other chemicals may have the same effect.

Thus any specimen of semen that shows either a marked reduction in volume or in sperm motility may simply be the result of poor production and handling prior to its arrival in the hospital.

Numbers of specimens that may be sent for analysis

Certainly in the management of infertility in the male, a reasonably accurate evaluation of the fertility status of the patient can usually only be achieved by assessing at least three samples of semen. As men may show cyclical changes in sperm production and as factors such as stress or even minor illness can have profound effects on semen quality, the laboratory may well be asked to report on several semen specimens from a single patient.

From the above, it can be seen that great care must be taken both by the clinician and by the laboratory to ensure that semen specimens are an accurate reflection of the patient's fertility and are not rendered invalid by stress, abnormal or incomplete ejaculation or by the action of physical or chemical damage during their transport to the laboratory. From the outset, it should now be clear that the analysis of semen does not simply consist of counting sperm. One important and most helpful role that the scientific staff can play in this respect is to demonstrate the presence of artifactual anomalies in semen. Each part of the examination of semen will now be studied in more detail.

References

Eliasson, R. (1965) Effect of frequent ejaculations on the composition of the human seminal plasma. *Journal of Reproduction and Fertility* **9**, 331–6.

Mortimer, D., Templeton, A. A., Lenton, E. A. & Coleman, R. A. (1982) Influence of abstinence and ejaculation-to-analysis delay on semen analysis parameters of suspected infertile men. *Archives of Andrology* **8,** 251–6.

6

Physical properties of Semen

An examination of the physical characteristics of seminal fluid make up an important part of the analysis of semen. How these features are assessed will now be described.

Volume of semen

The first step in the performance of a semen analysis is the estimation of the volume of the ejaculate. The volume of the semen specimen should *always* be measured as it is a very important sign of many disturbances within the genital tract. Even in azoospermic semen (where semen contains no sperm), a knowledge of the seminal volume can be most helpful. As will be shown later, the total number of sperm in an ejaculate should be calculated and for this, of course, the volume must have been measured. The presence of a low volume ejaculate may also be an important pointer to the presence of an incomplete specimen.

The suffix *spermia* denotes 'relating to seminal fluid' and not to spermatozoa. Changes in the volume of the semen are known by several names. *Aspermia* means the total absence of ejaculate and this is a rare phenomenon. The word aspermia is often used (quite wrongly) to mean the absence of spermatozoa in semen for which the correct word is *azoospermia*. A reduction in the volume of the ejaculate can be described by the word *oligospermia* which is also frequently (again quite incorrectly) used to describe sperm numbers. Because of this confusion, the word *hypospermia* is often used to describe a low volume ejaculate. The very rare phenomenon of increased semen volume is known as *hyperspermia* (Table 6.1).

There are many causes of infertility that are associated with a low volume ejaculate. As the majority of the seminal fluid comes from the seminal vesicles or prostate, abnormalities of these glands such as infective and inflammatory disorders will reduce their secretory powers and thus result in oligospermia. Reduction in secretion from the

Table 6.1. The terms used to describe the volume of an ejaculate

'spermia'	Suffix relating to semen
Aspermia	Absence of semen
Oligospermia/ Hypospermia	Reduced volume of semen i.e., <2ml
Hyperspermia	Increased volume of semen i.e., >10 ml

accessory glands will thus produce 'artifactual' concentrations of sperm. The condition of congenital absence of the vas deferentia is almost always associated with absence of the seminal vesicles. Such patients as these will have low volume semen which contains no sperm and also no fructose (the sugar produced by the seminal vesicles).

Abnormalities of ejaculation may also result in oligospermia. Such problems may be the result of stress and nervousness in the patient but can also result from many neurological disorders such as those associated with diabetes mellitus, multiple sclerosis and spinal cord abnormalities. Ejaculation can also occur in a retrograde manner so that most of the semen ends up in the bladder, a phenomenon known as *retrograde ejaculation*. In this situation, only the secretions of the bulbo-urethral glands will end up in the semen container resulting in a very low volume ejaculate indeed. Adequate testosterone production is also needed for normal sexual function and thus changes in semen volume may also result from endocrine disorders.

Measurement of semen volume

The volume of semen can be measured in several ways, using either a graduated pipette, a 5–10 ml graduated cylinder or a 10 ml graduated centrifuge tube. It is very important to remember that this glassware must be scrupulously clean as otherwise artifactual damage to the motility of the sperm will occur. For this reason, the use of disposable plastic apparatus is recommended as there can be no contamination of such containers and it is also guaranteed to be free of water. Semen volume can also be determined accurately by weighing the semen in a standard container (Eliasson, 1971).

The normal volume of semen is often quoted to lie between 2 and 6 ml but volumes as low as 1 ml and as high as 10 ml may also be regarded as normal. The volume is usually reported to the clinician as the volume in millilitres to the nearest 0.1 ml.

Colour of seminal fluid

Semen is normally a grey-yellow opalescent fluid. Its opacity is due, for the most part, to its high protein content but is of course also produced by the many millions of spermatozoa as well as the cellular debris that is normally suspended within it. However there are a number of pathological processes that will change the colour of semen and it is important that the person analysing semen is aware of the causes of these colour changes.

Urine

Urine may occasionally contaminate semen and this may occur in men with disturbances of bladder neck function and ejaculation. Unlike that occurring in jaundice, the presence of even relatively large amounts of urine in semen only produces a faint yellow discolouration but its presence can often be easily detected by the consistancy of the semen and by the uriniferous odour of the semen sample. A high urea content of the sample may confirm the presence of urine.

Urine, however, has a direct and lethal effect on spermatozoa. Contact between spermatozoa and even small amounts of urine will result in sperm death (Crich & Jequier, 1978). Thus specimens of semen which have been contaminated with urine will contain sperm which are either very poorly motile or even completely immotile.

Blood

The discolouration of semen that can be produced by blood (a condition known as haematospermia) depends on both the amount of blood present relative to the seminal volume and also the age of the blood. Traces of fresh blood will colour semen pink. Where relatively larger amounts of blood are present, the semen may be bright red. In situations where bleeding has occurred into the genital tract some hours or even days previously, such old blood may colour the semen brown.

As the most major contributors to semen are the seminal vesicles and the prostate, these are the most likely but not the only sources of blood in semen. Infection of the seminal vesicles or prostate and in particular infection by tuberculosis, are the most common causes of haematospermia but in older men it may also occasionally be associated with prostatic carcinoma. Trauma or malignancy of the testes can also produce this abnormality. However, in a lot of patients the source of the blood is difficult to identify. Split ejaculates may be used in an attempt to demonstrate the source of the blood. In many patients the bleeding may only occur once and thus its origins cannot be traced. In other men, blood may appear in semen intermittently which also makes the identification of its source very difficult. In older patients the presence of cancer must be excluded. However in most young patients, the bleeding is nearly always associated with infection. Thus if any one fraction of a split ejaculate shows, even in the absence of blood, an excessive number of white cells, it is likely that it is this fraction of the ejaculate that has previously contained the blood.

Jaundice

Just as it will colour many other tissues and body fluids, bilirubin will also colour semen. In deep jaundice, the semen may be a very bright yellow. It is possible that the fact that the patient is jaundiced may not even be recorded on the card and thus the bright yellow colour of semen that occurs in men with jaundice may be quite startling to anyone analysing semen who is unaware of this phenomenon.

The presence of bilirubin in seminal fluid may, *per se*, have little effect on semen quality but the associated liver disease can severely disturb spermatogenesis and thus indirectly, and very profoundly, effect both the sperm count and the sperm motility.

pH of semen

The pH of semen can on occasions be of value to the clinician and should be recorded on each specimen.

The pH of normal fresh semen lies between 7.9 and 8.1. The pH should only be recorded on fresh semen as it may slowly fall as the specimen ages. The pH of semen is most easily measured using a pH paper with a range of 6.6–9.0 (Fig. 6.1). This is available in most laboratories. The use of a pH meter is unnecessary as such precision is not needed, and seminal fluid which is relatively viscous may produce blockage of the pH meter. It must be remembered that semen is a very powerful buffer as it contains large amounts of protein. However,

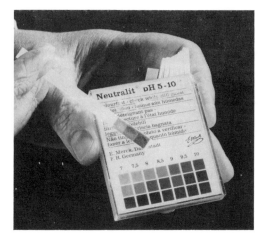

Fig. 6. 1. Litmus paper of the type used to test the pH of semen.

inflammatory conditions, particularly of the prostate or seminal vesicles, may alter the pH of semen and this information may be of value to the clinician.

Liquefaction of semen

In most mammals semen is ejaculated in a liquid form. In some species such as the bull and the ram, it remains liquid. After ejaculation, pig semen forms a gel while in the rodents it forms a firm coagulum often referred to as a 'plug' (Mann, 1964). In the human, semen forms a gel-like clot after ejaculation but within about 5–20 minutes, liquefaction of this clot has occurred.

The coagulation of human semen is dependent on the presence of a fibrinogen-like substrate manufactured by the seminal vesicles which is acted upon by the enzyme vesiculase produced by the prostate. Absence of the seminal vesicular or of prostatic secretions may therefore be associated with absence of coagulation of the semen. Breakdown of the clot and the associated fibrin takes place as the result of the activities of a series of proteolytic enzymes secreted by the prostate and these include proteases, pepsinogen and amylase, and even hyaluronidase. Further peptide breakdown can occur due to the concomitant presence of transaminase enzymes. Therefore both clotting and liquefaction are induced, at least in part, by the secretions of the prostate.

Absence of liquefaction (and thus the containment of the sperm within the gel) may cause infertility (Amelar, 1962) but frequently impairment of liquefaction is associated with normal fertility. However the possible absence of a prostatic component in the ejaculate may be of importance diagnostically. For this reason, abnormalities of liquefaction should be noted during the performance of a semen analysis.

Assessment of liquefaction

Liquefaction of the clot should be complete within 20 minutes of ejaculation. Thus if a specimen of semen is brought into the hospital from outside, liquefaction should, by this time, be complete.

Liquefaction is usually assessed visually. Unliquefied semen forms a gel like coagulum. Partially liquefied semen may contain many small gel like clots and in fully liquefied semen no such clots are seen and the semen appears completely fluid.

It is, however, possible to measure the speed of liquefaction in comparison with that of a normal donor by using the third fraction of a split ejaculate (Tauber *et al.*, 1973). The third fraction of a split ejaculate liquefies very slowly and liquefaction is not usually complete for 1–2 hours. The third fraction is placed in a nylon mesh net suspended in a 2–3 ml graduated tube. The coagulum cannot pass through the net but after liquefaction the seminal fluid will pass through the net into the tube. The speed and also the rate of liquefaction of the 'slowly lysing' fraction of semen can then be readily compared with that of a normal donor. The end point is when liquefaction is complete and the nylon bag is empty. It is also possible to compare the effect of one fraction on another in terms of both coagulation and liquefaction and thus attempt to diagnose the accessory organ that may be the cause of the patient's non-liquefaction of semen.

Abnormalities of liquefaction must not be confused with abnormalities of viscosity which will be discussed in the next section. It is very important to differentiate the two.

Treatment of unliquefied semen

In cases of infertility which are associated with unliquefied semen (and these cases are rare), treatment of the semen with proteolytic enzymes which lyse the clot may be undertaken. Artificial insemination of this treated semen can then be employed in an attempt to achieve pregnancy.

A variety of enzymes have been described for use on unliquefied semen. The most commonly used enzyme is alpha-amylase (Bunge & Sherman, 1954). The enzyme alpha-amylase is used as a 0.2% solution and 5–10 drops may be added to an ejaculate of average volume. Other enzymes can also be used in similar concentrations and these include alpha-chymotrypsin, lysozyme (Hirschhausser & Eliasson, 1972) and hyaluronidase (Amelar, 1962). If excessive quantities or concentrations of the enzymes are used on semen, their proteolytic activity may tend to damage sperm by digestion of the cell membranes. Thus the minimum amount of enzyme that will liquefy the ejaculate is optimal for the treatment of this disorder.

It is important, however, to state that non-liquefaction in semen *must* be differentiated from semen that is simply excessively viscous.

Viscosity of semen

The viscosity of the seminal fluid may vary considerably both between different patients and also between different semen samples from the same individual. There is some evidence that increased viscosity may be associated with infertility. However, thick hyperviscid semen does make accurate counting of sperm more difficult and causes the introduction of errors into a semen analysis.

Normal viscosity is defined as that which will allow semen to be poured drop by drop out of a container (Eliasson, 1971). Viscosity can also be quantified by measuring the time it will take for 1 drop of semen to leave a standard pipette. The diameter of the pipette will greatly influence the flow rate of the semen through it and thus these pipettes must be of a fixed size. Usually a capillary tube of 10 cm in length and which contains 0.1 ml of semen may be used, the pipettes having previously been standardized using a substance such as silicon oil. Using this technique, viscosity is assessed and only a very small volume of semen need be used in this test. However, with experience, degrees of viscosity can be fairly easily assessed by its ease of aspiration up a Pasteur pipette.

Hyperviscosity as a cause of infertility

The exact role that hyperviscosity of semen may play in infertility is very poorly understood and much work is needed to clarify this problem. It has been suggested that hyperviscid semen may fail to coat the cervix and may too easily drain out of the vagina after intercourse. Theoretically, a very viscid seminal fluid might also impair the ability of the spermatozoa contained within it to escape into the cervical mucus. However, sperm from many hyperviscid semen samples show no difficulty in entering cervical mucus at microscopy. It is the experience of the authors that many hyperviscid semen specimens are indeed normally fertile. At least 10% of post vasectomy semen specimens are hyperviscid, the great majority of which must have come from men of known fertility (Crich, unpublished). Hyperviscid semen samples also occur from donors to an AID programme and judging by their ability to produce pregnancies, give no reason to believe that such semen is of reduced fertility.

Treatment of excessively viscous semen

Excessively viscous semen can be made more fluid in a number of different ways. The most frequently described method of rendering hyperviscid semen more fluid is by passing it down a wide bore needle (gauge 18 or 23). However, during their passage down the needle the sperm may be damaged, thus affecting the potential fertility of the semen. Reduction of viscosity may also be achieved by mixing the viscid semen with sperm-free seminal fluid from another patient. It must be remembered that sperm antibody interactions could occur in these circumstances and reduce the fertility of the semen undergoing such treatment.

The whole subject of seminal hyperviscosity clearly needs better evaluation. In the meantime the presence of hyperviscid semen must be reported at a semen analysis.

References

Amelar, R. D. (1962) Coagulation, liquefaction and viscosity of human semen. *Journal of Urology* **87**, 187–90.

Bunge, R. G. & Sherman, J. K. (1954) Liquefaction of human semen by alpha-amylase. *Fertility and Sterility* **5**, 353–6.

Crich, J. P., & Jequier, A. M. (1978) Infertility in men with retrograde ejaculation: The action of urine on sperm motility and a simple method for achieving antegrade ejaculation. *Fertility and Sterility* **30**, 572–6.

Eliasson, R. (1971) Standards for the investigation of human semen. *Andrologie* **3**, 49–64.

Hirschhausser, C. & Eliasson, R. (1972) Origin and possible function of muramidase (lysozyme) in human seminal plasma. *Life Sciences* **11** (Pt. 2), 149–54.

Mann, T. (1964) *The Biochemistry of Semen*, pp. 76–8. John Wiley and Sons Inc., New York.

Tauber, P. F., Zaneveld, L. J. D., Propping, D. & Schumacher, G. F. B. (1973) Biochemical studies on the lysis of human split ejaculates. *Biology of Reproduction* **9**, Abstract, 62.

7

Sperm Count

The determination of the numbers of spermatozoa in semen forms an important part of any semen analysis. Several terms are used to describe sperm numbers in semen. The *sperm concentration* describes the number of sperm in millions that are present per unit volume of seminal fluid. The unit volume generally used is the millilitre but in some centres the sperm concentration is now reported as the number of spermatozoa per litre. However, the sperm concentration takes no account of the total number of sperm in an ejaculate which is probably a better indication of fertility potential than is the sperm concentration alone. For example, a concentration of 10 million sperm per ml in a semen sample of 5 ml in volume will provide a total of 50 million sperm in the ejaculate; while a semen specimen containing 20 million sperm per ml but totalling only 0.5 ml in volume will produce an ejaculate containing a total of only 10 million sperm. Thus in reporting the number of spermatozoa in semen, the volume must be taken into account. The *total sperm count* is the total number of spermatozoa in an ejaculate and is obtained by multiplying the sperm concentration by the volume of the sample of semen. It is essential to include *both* these values in a report.

Several more generalized terms are used to describe both sperm concentration and sperm count: *azoospermia* describes a total absence of spermatozoa in semen. The word aspermia is frequently (but quite wrongly) used in place of azoospermia. *Oligozoospermia* refers to a reduced number of sperm in semen and is usually used to describe a sperm concentration of less than 20 million sperm per ml or a total sperm count of less than 50 million spermatozoa. The word oligospermia is also frequently (but quite wrongly) used in place of oligozoospermia. *Polyzoospermia* denotes an increased number of spermatozoa in semen and usually refers to a sperm concentration in excess of 350 million per ml.

Methods of measuring sperm concentration

Spermatozoa are very small structures and a good microscope is essential in any laboratory performing semen analyses. Phase contrast microscopy is very useful indeed and, as will be discussed later, is of particular value when assessing the motility and morphology of the sperm. Although phase contrast optics are relatively expensive, they are also of particular help to those who are inexperienced in semen analysis because phase contrast makes the identification, particularly of abnormal sperm, that much more accurate. In the absence of phase contrast, a microscope with good definition and capable of a magnification of at least × 400 is essential. It is now of value to consider the methods available for determining sperm concentration.

It must be remembered that as only an aliquot of the semen specimen will be used to assess sperm concentration, it is essential the specimen is *well mixed*. Dead sperm will tend to sink to the bottom of the specimen jar and thus are easy to exclude from the estimation. Gentle rotation of the jar containing the specimen or careful application of the container to a slow vortex is usually sufficient to provide adequate mixing.

Visual assessment

The application of a drop of well mixed semen to a clean glass slide under a lightly-applied glass coverslip will allow visualization of the sperm in a specimen of semen. Those who are experienced in seminal fluid analysis are frequently able to make quite an accurate assessment of sperm concentrations in this way. Such a method, often familiarly called 'eye-balling', must not be employed by the inexperienced or when the semen analysis is being used to assess response to treatment, or more particularly, as part of a research project. Such quick visual assessments are, however, very useful as an interim or quick report should this be necessary. Many clinicians like to give their patients at least some idea of the outcome of the semen analysis before the patient leaves the clinic. For these purposes, visual assessment is of some value.

Visual assessment of sperm concentration is also used in determining the need for dilution of semen prior to performing the formal estimation of sperm concentration.

The improved Neubauer Counting Chamber (Haemocytometer)

In the majority of laboratories where semen analyses are carried out, it is this counting chamber that is most frequently used. The advantage of this chamber is that it is cheap and is freely available in all pathology laboratories. Its disadvantage, however, is that it is time-consuming to use and, because of the necessity for dilution of the semen, it is a method subject to error. The new improved Neubauer Counting Chamber is made up of two grids lying on either side of a central trough. Thus it is simple to perform duplicate counts on each diluted semen sample. However, the semen must be diluted first.

Dilution of the semen

With experience, the initial visual assessment of sperm concentration as described above, will allow the correct dilution to be made prior to the formal counting in the haemocytometer (Fig. 7.1). The usual dilution of semen needed for its analysis in the Neubauer Counting Chamber is 1 in 20 or 1 part of semen to 19 parts of diluent (vol/vol). Thus a 50 µl aliquot of *well mixed* semen is mixed with 950 µl of diluent. For semen samples containing very low numbers of sperm, a 1 in 10 dilution may be used instead. Conversely in patients with a very high sperm concentration, a 1 in 50 dilution may also be employed.

All dilutions are best carried out using an automatic pipette. A white cell pipette is too inaccurate for this procedure and should *never* be used. The diluent employed varies from laboratory to laboratory but most diluents are designed to immobilize sperm and thus facilitate counting. The most frequently used diluent is a buffered 3.5% formal saline (Table 7.1). If this is not available, tap water will also kill sperm and thus will suffice as a diluent. However, it must be remembered that tap water causes coiling of the sperm tails and other distortions. Thus morphological assessment of sperm must *not* be performed on diluted semen containing immobilized sperm, most especially when the diluent used is tap water.

Staining of the sperm

Staining of the sperm can be achieved by the addition of Gentian violet (to produce a 0.5% solution) to the buffered formal saline and this may

Chapter 7

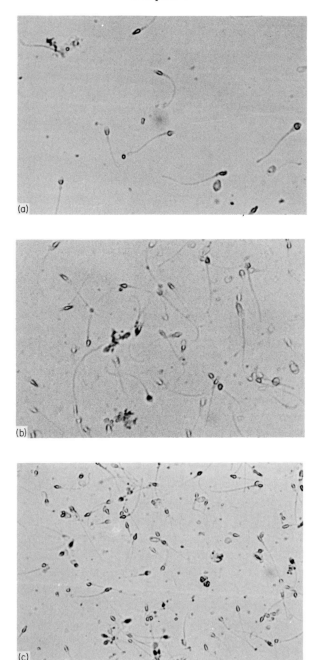

Fig. 7.1. Wet preparation of semen which were subsequently shown to contain sperm at concentrations of (a) 10, (b) 50 and (c) 100 million per ml. (Original magnification × 1600.)

Table 7.1. The formulation of buffered 3.5% formal saline for use as a semen diluent

Buffered Formal Saline	
Na H CO$_3$	5.0 Grams
35% Formalin	1 ml
Distilled water	to produce final volume of 100 ml

To produce a stain, 5 ml of saturated aqueous Gentian violet may be included in the final volume.

aid their identification from other cells present in semen. The use of a stain may therefore be of particular help to the inexperienced analyst of semen but it will of course also stain all the other cellular debris in the semen.

The aliquot of semen and the diluent are mixed in a small tube. The most commonly used tubes for this purpose are LP3 tubes or some other small glass test tube which can be applied safely to a vortex.

Preparation of the counting chamber

For use in a semen analysis, the improved Neubauer Counting Chamber (Fig. 7.2) must be very clean. Prior to its use, it should be

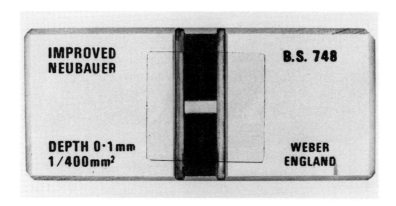

Fig. 7.2. The improved Neubauer Counting Chamber.

Chapter 7

washed with its coverslip in distilled water and both must be carefully dried with a lens tissue. It is very important that the counting chamber is free of grease.

To prepare the chamber for use, the clean, dry coverslip is pressed onto the glass base, and using the thumbs, is slid gently forward, over the counting grids. Pressure is maintained on the coverslip until all the air between the glass is excluded when the bi-refringent rings, often known as Newton's Rings, become clearly visible. Only when these rings are seen is the chamber ready for use. Absence of bi-refringent rings means usually that the coverslip is insecurely applied to the chamber.

It is now time to apply the diluted semen to the chamber. It must at this point be remembered that all the sperm in the diluent are dead and will tend to sink to the bottom of their container. Careful mixing of the semen and diluent is *very important* and application of the tube containing the diluted semen to a slow vortex will ensure adequate mixing at this stage.

Using a Pasteur pipette, a small drop of the well mixed diluted semen is now applied to the outer edges of the coverslip on each side of the central trough (Fig. 7.3). The diluted semen will now spread out

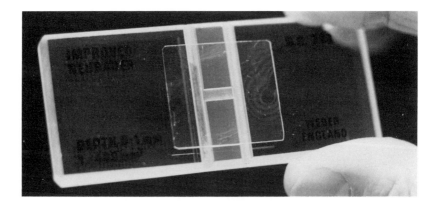

Fig. 7.3. The correct method of application of the semen–diluent mixture to the outer edge of an improved Neubauer Counting Chamber. The bifurnagent rings are visible.

under the coverslip to fill each section of the counting chamber. Each chamber is then viewed microscopically usually at a magnification of $\times 200$ using a $\times 20$ objective and a $\times 10$ eyepiece.

Estimation of sperm concentration

Viewed down the microscope, each counting chamber is made up of 9 large squares which cover a total of 9 mm^2 (Fig. 7.4). For the semen analysis, only the central large square is used.

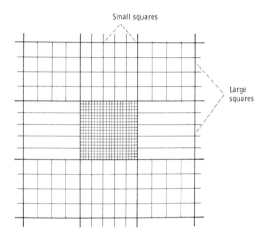

Small squares

Large squares

Fig. 7.4. One of the grids in an improved Neubauer Counting Chamber.

The central large square is subdivided into 25 smaller squares. Of these small squares only 5 are selected for counting sperm. It is traditional that the 4 corner squares and the central square are used but of course any 5 squares can be selected provided they are not adjoining squares. The number of sperm within each selected small square are now counted. It is usual that any sperm touching the outer margins of two of the four sides of the square are excluded from the count and those sperm touching the remaining margins of the squares are included in the count. In this way, the number of sperm (each accurately identified) in 5 small squares, are totalled. It is important to remember that germinal cells and loose tails must *not* be included in the count. The count is then repeated in the opposite chamber. The sperm concentration may then be calculated in the following way:

Each large square = 1 mm^2

As each large square contains 25 small squares then:

Each small square = $\frac{1}{25}$ = 0.04 mm^2

5 small squares = 0.2 mm^2

Number of sperm/mm^2 = 'sperm count' × 5.

∴ sperm count/µl × 10 = concentration of sperm/µl of diluted semen (to account for chamber depth)

If the dilution was $\frac{1}{20}$, then sperm concentration/µl of neat semen = count/µl × 20

Therefore sperm concentration/ml = count/ml × 1000

A perhaps more simple method of calculating the sperm concentration is given below:

Count (sperm in 5 small squares) × 20 (dilution)

× 5($\frac{1}{5}$ mm^2 is area in which sperm are counted)

× 10 (depth in µm of counting chamber) × 1000 (to convert mm^3 to ml) = Number of sperm/ml

A calculation is made in this way for the sperm counted on each side of the chamber and the results expressed as a mean.

For good precision and accuracy a total of 200 spermatozoa should be counted and if this total is not achieved, then the dilution of the semen must be adjusted accordingly. It is also good practice to perform these counts using two aliquots of semen which have been separately diluted. The value obtained from these two separately diluted aliquots of semen must not differ by more than 15%. If these principles are adhered to, then precise and reliable estimates of sperm concentration will be obtained. Such estimates are valid not only in the clinical management of male infertility but also as an adjunct to many a clinical research project. Such accuracy is essential not only to judge fertility but also for any research project where semen quality may need to be judged retrospectively.

The Makler Counting Chamber

Unlike the Neubauer Haemocytometer, the Makler Counting Chamber* has been specifically designed (Makler, 1980) for use with semen (Fig. 7.5). Although it is relatively expensive, the ease and the

* Available from Sefi Medical Instruments – US suppliers Zygotek™ Systems Inc., 130 Maple St., Suite 232, Springfield, Mass 01103.

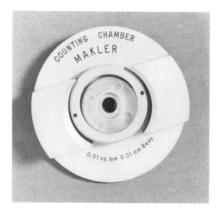

Fig. 7.5. The Makler Counting Chamber.

speed with which it can be used to estimate sperm concentration makes it, in the authors' opinion, highly cost effective.

The main advantage of the Makler Counting Chamber is that no dilution of the semen is needed except when the sperm concentration is exceptionally high. This saves time and reduces error. The second advantage of the Makler Chamber is that an assessment of motility, forward progression and to some extent of morphology can be made at the same time as the count.

The chamber itself consists of two parts (Fig. 7.6). The main lower part is made up of flat metal ring base and two metal 'handles'. On the

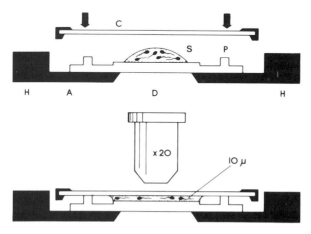

Fig. 7.6. A diagrammatic representation of the Makler Counting Chamber (reproduced by kind permission of Dr A. Makler and Sefi-Medical Instruments Ltd.).

upper surface of this ring is fixed a glass disc on which the semen is placed. Arising from the edge of this ring are four quartz coated pins which rise up 10 μm above the surface of the central glass disc. The upper part of the chamber forms the coverglass and consists of a disc of glass held in a metal ring. On the lower surface of this cover glass is marked a 1 mm² grid which is subdivided into 100 squares each 0.1 × 0.1 mm² in size (Fig. 7.7). Thus when the cover glass is placed on the four quartz coated pins, the space bounded by the two surfaces and 10 of the small squares is 0.001 mm³ (or 1 millionth of a ml). Thus the number of sperm counted in 10 squares is the same number × 10⁶ that are present in 1 ml of semen. No difficult calculations are therefore needed to determine the sperm concentrations.

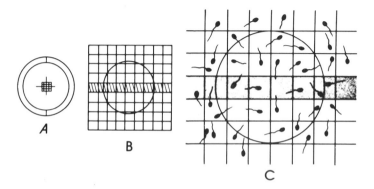

Fig. 7.7. The grid of the Makler Counting Chamber (reproduced by kind permission of Dr A. Makler and Sefi-Medical Instruments Ltd.).

Preparation of the Makler Counting Chamber

In the performance of the sperm count using the Makler Chamber, as with the Neubauer Counting Chamber, it is very important that the Makler Chamber is clean. This is best achieved using distilled water and by drying the chamber and coverglass with a lens tissue. As the depth of the chamber must be accurately maintained, it is important first to place the coverglass on the base and test that Newton's rings will appear around the four supporting corner pins. The cover glass is then removed.

A *small* drop of semen is now placed on the central glass disc of the lower part of the chamber (Fig. 7.8). It is best if the semen does not fill

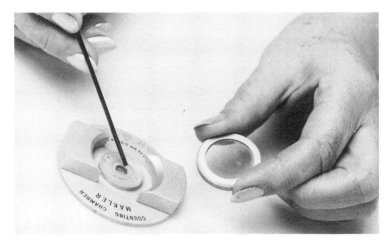

Fig. 7.8. The application of semen to a Makler Counting Chamber (reproduced by kind permission of Dr A. Makler and Sefi-Medical Instruments Ltd.).

this area and it is of course important to avoid the presence of air bubbles. Only a small amount of practice is required for this manoeuvre to be done successfully. The cover glass is then placed over the semen, again looking for the appearance of the birefringent rings. This manoeuvre will ensure the automatic spread of the drop of semen to a thickness of 10 μm. The chamber is now lifted by its handles onto the microscope stage and viewed using phase contrast optics for preference at a minimum magnification of × 200. It is best to use a × 20 objective and a × 10 eyepiece.

On examining the semen through the grid, it is first important to ensure that the sperm are evenly distributed: an uneven distribution of sperm means that the original sample was inadequately mixed. The sperm examined in the Makler are undiluted and are therefore motile. One may think that this makes the count more difficult but the main advantage of the layer of semen present under the grid of a Makler Counting Chamber is that it is only one sperm deep. Thus no adjustment to the focus need be made during the count and the sperm content of the squares to be counted is easily visualized. If the sperm are in high concentration and are therefore difficult to count, they can be immobilized. This is best done by putting an aliquot of the semen into a test tube and incubating it for 5 minutes at 50–60°C. Semen so treated can then be used for the estimation of the sperm concentration without the need for dilution and all the errors that this involves. However, in semen where the sperm are in very great concentration, dilution may be necessary.

The calculation of the sperm concentration is easy. As 10 squares is equal to 0.001 mm^3, then the number of sperm in 10 squares equals the sperm concentration in millions per ml. It is important to repeat this count using another strip of 10 squares and also to repeat the whole of this duplicate count on another aliquot of the semen.

Thus using the Makler makes the estimation of the sperm concentration very simple indeed. As will be seen later, it can also be used to assess sperm motility as well as their morphology.

The chamber is cleaned between analyses by washing in distilled water. The apparatus is best dried using lens tissue and final cleaning can be achieved using a camel hair brush.

The Horwell Fertility Counting Chamber

This counting chamber was also designed specifically for semen analyses by Horwell*. It is much cheaper than the Makler, though based on similar principles. No dilution is needed and the chamber depth is also 10 μm. The grid also consists of 100 squares and the counting is performed in the same way as with the grid on the Makler Counting Chamber. Despite their price these specialized counting chambers save a great deal of time and should certainly be recommended for use in any busy laboratory that may perform many semen analyses in a day.

Sperm counting based on the laser principle

There are being developed at the present time, a number of new methods of estimating sperm concentration. One of these involves the use of laser light. From the deflection of a beam of laser light, a computer can determine not only the sperm concentration but also the sperm motility as well as the presence or absence of forward progression. Such apparatus is of course still very expensive, but one feels sure that in the future methods like this will be in common use.

* Details available from A. R. Horwell, 73 Maygrove Rd, W. Hampstead, London NW6 2BP.

Expression of results

Precision is vital in most laboratory procedures and in semen analysis precision is more than usually important. The most important factor in determining good results is adequate mixing and *very careful* dilution techniques. Each estimation of sperm concentration must be performed in duplicate and if dilution is used, it must be performed in duplicate using two specially diluted aliquots of semen.

The values obtained from two dilutions should show a coefficient of variation of not more than 15%. The sperm concentrations so obtained should be averaged and quoted on the report as the sperm concentration per ml. The total sperm count is reported as the average sperm concentration multiplied by the volume of the semen sample.

Obtaining a permanent visual record of sperm concentrations

Although this is not necessary for routine work, a photograph may be taken of a counting chamber grid as a useful record of research purposes. An ordinary black and white photograph is usually adequate, but of course one must have a camera with the appropriate attachment to the microscope. If even more capital expenditure is possible, a record of both count and motility may be obtained using a video camera and recorder.

References

Makler, A. (1980) The improved ten-micrometer chamber for rapid sperm count and motility evaluation. *Fertility and Sterility* **33**, 337–8.

8

Assessment of Sperm Movement

In order to achieve fertilization, a sperm must not only be able to move but be capable of movement that results in forward progression. Forward progression is often also known as *progressive activity*. Such forward movement is needed not only for a sperm to enter and pass through the female genital tract but also for it to penetrate the coverings of the oocyte and achieve fertilization. Although sperm transport through the genital tract may be aided by the ciliary action of the epithelial lining of the uterus and fallopian tubes, vigorous forward movement of the sperm would appear nevertheless to be essential for fertility. Thus the more sperm in a semen sample that are demonstrating both movement and forward progression, the greater will be the fertility potential of that semen. Assessment of sperm movement both quantitatively as well as qualitatively is an important part of a semen analysis. Not only must the number of moving sperm be estimated but the quality of their movement must also be assessed.

Terms used to describe abnormalities of sperm movement are *asthenozoospermia*, which describes an absence or a marked reduction in sperm movement. As abnormalities of sperm movement are commonly associated with a reduction in sperm numbers, the word *oligoasthenozoospermia* is often used to describe this type of abnormality in semen.

Sperm movement is a complex process. As the result of contractions of the fibres contained in the axoneme, a 'paddle' movement is induced. The head turns its flat surface from side to side while undulations of the tail cause the sperm to move forward. These undulations of the tail occur in two planes. The amplitude of the waves of tail movement is greater in the flat plane of the head than that occurring in the narrow plane of the head (Fig. 8.1).

If sperm are correctly illuminated during microscopy and especially if phase contrast optics are used, light is reflected off the flat surface of each sperm head to produce a spot of light which is also known as the

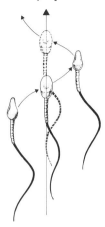

Fig. 8.1. A diagrammatic representation of the paddle movement made by spermatozoa and which results in forward progression.

'light reflex'. As the sperm head performs its paddle movement, the light reflex is temporarily lost until the flat surface of the sperm head becomes visible again. An absence of the turning 'on and off' of the light reflex is a sign that sperm movement is abnormal.

Assessment of sperm movement

In many laboratories, the motility and forward progression of sperm is still assessed in a very subjective way and in most instances the results quoted on a report are little more than a 'guesstemate' albeit often a fairly good one. As counting motile sperm is really not that arduous, it is best to use methods that give reasonably repeatable results.

Quantitative assessment

If a sperm is showing any movement at all (and it does not matter whether that movement is normal or abnormal) the sperm is said to be motile. For the purposes of a semen analysis, sperm motility may be recorded as the 'percentage motility', that is, the percentage of the total sperm that are showing movement. It is best if the numbers of motile sperm per ml is also calculated and recorded on the report as the 'motile sperm count':

$$\text{Motile Sperm Count} = \frac{\text{Sperm conc. ml} \times \% \text{ motility} \times \text{semen vol.}}{100}$$

The estimation of percentage motility must be performed soon after the production of the semen sample (depending on when the sample was delivered to the laboratory) and such assessment should be repeated at 3 hours and at 6 hours after production. Each estimation of motility should be performed in duplicate and the mean result recorded on the report. As with any other estimation, the coefficient of variation between duplicates should not exceed 15%.

Qualitative assessment

The quality of sperm movement is determined, in most laboratories, using methods which are subjective.

The quality of sperm movement is usually graded according to the type of movement made by the largest proportion of the total sperm. The grading used can be numerical or descriptive but is probably best described using phrases that are easily understood by all clinicians. If numerals are used, sperm movement is graded from 0–4 (Table 8.1). This method has the advantage of simplicity but will not be easily understood by those clinicians who infrequently interpret semen analyses. Descriptive words such as 'poor', 'moderate' or 'excellent' are more helpful but a phrase that fully describes sperm movement, for example, 'Total absence of forward progression' or 'Good forward progression' is the most helpful of all.

Table 8.1. Methods of describing the quality of the forward movement (progressive activity) of sperm for a semen analysis

Definition	Description
0 — None	An absence of forward progression
1 — Poor	Weak or sluggish forward progression
2 — Moderate	Definite forward progression
3 — Good	Good forward movement with progression
4 — Excellent	Vigorous rapid forward progression

Methods used to assess sperm movement

There are two main ways in which both the quantity and the quality of sperm motility can be estimated.

Slide technique

This simple method is probably the most frequent way in which sperm motility is assessed. It must be remembered however that each sperm needs a minimum of 10 μm of depth in order to maintain unimpeded movement. Thus normal sperm lying on a slide under a coverslip that has been too forcefully applied will not be able to move. Artifactual abnormalities in movement may therefore occur.

A drop of well mixed undiluted semen is placed on the surface of a warm, dry and very clean microscope slide. On top of the semen is placed a coverslip. (The coverslip must not be pressed down onto the glass slide or it may well impede the movement of the sperm.) The slide is allowed to rest on the bench or on the microscope stage until all 'streaming' of the sperm has stopped. The drop of semen is then viewed at a magnification of around × 250–400, preferably using a microscope equipped with phase contrast. Both the motile and the immotile sperm are counted in at least 5 separate microscopic fields. A minimum of around 200 sperm should be counted. The percentage motility is calculated from the mean values.

The quality of the sperm movement is then graded. If any very abnormal movement, for example, circular movement, is seen it should be recorded on the report.

Counting chamber

If one is fortunate enough to have the use of a purpose-made counting chamber such as the Makler or the Horwell Chambers, then the percentage motility and also an assessment of the quality of sperm movement can be performed at the same time as the sperm count. These chambers also have a depth of 10 μm and thus impedance of sperm movement cannot occur. The same number of sperm must be counted and the motile sperm present are expressed as a percentage of the total. Similarly a qualitative grading of sperm is made in the same way as with the slide method.

Photography and its use in assessing sperm movement

Photomicrography and its application to semen may appear at first sight to be an expensive and perhaps not very relevant approach to fertility assessment of sperm. It does however now have a very important role to play in the analysis of semen. There are a number of ways in which photography can be applied to semen which will supply information about sperm movement and sperm function that cannot be obtained any other way.

Stroboscopic multiple exposure

This technique provides an excellent way of analysing sperm movement. It was first described by Makler (1978) and employs pulses of light to produce a multiple exposed photograph of a sperm moving across a field. For this a Makler Counting Chamber must be used in order that the field of view is only one sperm deep and each sperm stays in focus. A circular metal plate fixed to a turntable (an old gramophone turntable serves very well) is placed between the light source and the microscope table. Into this circular disc are cut 6 slits which are constructed so as to produce 6 exposures during one second. Using appropriate film, a photograph consisting of six 'exposures' of moving sperm is obtained (Fig. 8.2). The straightness or otherwise of the forward progression of sperm can now be clearly visualized, charted, measured and stored as a permanent record.

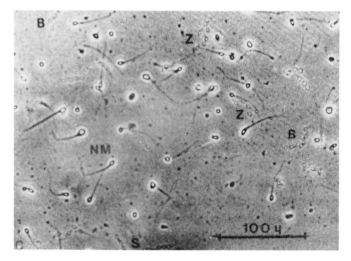

Fig. 8.2. A multiple exposed photograph of spermatozoa in semen. The moving sperm in these photographs produce 'chains' of heads, each head representing one of the exposures. The immotile sperm are seen as a single well exposed image. (Photograph reproduced by kind permission from Makler, A. (1980) Use of the Elaborated Multiple Exposure Photography (MEP) Method in Routine Sperm Motility Analysis and for Research Purposes. *Fertility and Sterility* **33**, 160–66).

Prolonged exposure and measurement of sperm velocity

A sperm's progress across a field can also be charted using a prolonged exposure line. In a method described by Milligan *et al.* (1978), sperm are photographed using an exposure time of 2 seconds. Such a photograph will show the tracks made by the sperm head across a field (Fig. 8.3). Using a graticule as an internal standard, the lengths of these tracks may be measured and thus the velocity of the forwardly moving sperm can be calculated. It would seem that velocity of sperm correlates fairly well with potential fertility. The mean velocity of fertile spermatozoa appears to be around 25–40 μm/second depending on the temperature of the semen sample.

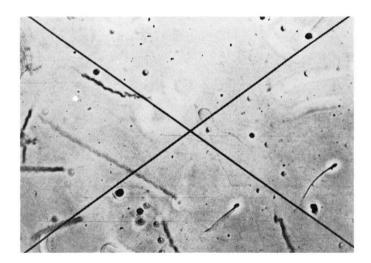

Fig. 8.3. A prolonged exposure of semen containing motile sperm. In this photograph, the motile sperm are seen as continuous linear images (Milligan *et al.*, 1978). The diagonal graticule is used in the calculation of sperm velocity.

Prolonged exposure photography has also recently been shown to be valuable in predicting fertility in another way. Using dark ground illumination, and an exposure time of one second, Aitkin *et al.* (1985) have recently demonstrated that the width of the path taken by the sperm head during forward movement is important in determining potential fertility, that is, a critical width of the path taken by the head of a sperm is needed before the sperm can penetrate cervical mucus. This particular feature of sperm movement cannot be assessed in any way other than by photography and thus this technique may be of great value in the analysis of semen.

Photomicrography is also an excellent way of storing information about a semen analysis. If a grid of a counting chamber is photographed a record of sperm concentration can be obtained. Using multiple or prolonged exposure, a record of sperm concentration and of both quantitative and qualitative motility will be achieved.

Laser light

Recently, laser light and the Doppler shift has been used to determine sperm numbers as well as to produce an estimate of both quantitative and qualitative sperm motility (Jouannet *et al.*, 1977). Such apparatus which is used in conjunction with a computer is therefore very expensive but may one day be of value in the performance of semen analysis.

Videomicrography

Use is now being made of the video recorder (Katz & Overstreet, 1981). By fitting a television camera to the microscope, one may now analyse sperm movement as has never been possible before. By using specially adapted fast forward video recorders, one can obtain slow motion pictures of sperm, many aspects of which can be analysed with the help of computers. Video micrographic analysis of sperm movement is a new subject but one which we will hear a lot more of in the future.

References

Aitken, R. J., Sutton, M., Warner, P. & Richardson, D. W. (1985) Relationship between the movement characteristics of human spermatozoa and their ability to penetrate cervical mucus and zona-free hamster oocytes. *Journal of Reproduction and Fertility* **73**, 441–9.

Jouannet, P., Valochine, B., Dequent, P., Semes, C. & David, E. (1977) Light scattering determination of various characteristic parameters of spermatozoa motility in a seris of human sperm. *Andrologia* **9**, 36–49.

Katz, D. F. & Overstreet, J. W. (1981) Sperm motility assessed by videomicrography. *Fertility and Sterility* **35**, 188–93.

Makler, A. (1978) A new multiple exposure photography method for objective human spermatozoal motility determination. *Fertility and Sterility* **30**, 192–9.

Milligan, M. P., Harris, S. J. & Dennis, K. J. (1978) The effect of temperature on the velocity of human spermatozoa as measured by time-lapse photography. *Fertility and Sterility* **30**, 592–4.

9

Assessment of Sperm Morphology

The identification of different types of abnormal spermatozoa in semen is a very important part of a semen analysis. The many structural abnormalities that may occur in sperm are known to be associated with infertility. Demonstration of their presence in a semen sample is of great importance in determining the potential fertility of that semen. An accurate assessment of sperm morphology is just as an important part of a semen analysis as is the sperm count.

It is at this point in the semen analysis that the presence of other cellular components of seminal fluid such as epithelial cells and most especially white blood cells (or pus cells) may be identified, as all these additional cellular elements in semen may have some bearing on the potential fertility of an ejaculate. It should also be remembered that it is possible on rare occasions to identify cells with malignant potential in the semen of infertile men and it is clearly important that such cells be positively identified (Crich, unpublished).

The morphology of a sperm can be assessed either by light microscopy or by the use of the electron microscope. The use of the latter method is time-consuming and the equipment very expensive but there are however a small number of patients in whom the examination of the sperm by transmission electron microscopy is very useful diagnostically. Such an examination provides information about the sperm that cannot be gained in any other way. However, the great majority of semen analyses can be carried out very satisfactorily using light microscopy alone.

The terms commonly used in relation to abnormalities in the morphology of spermatozoa are *teratozoospermia* and *teratoasthenozoospermia*. *Teratozoospermia* describes the presence of an increase in the numbers of morphologically abnormal sperm in a semen sample. As abnormal sperm often show poor or absent motility, the term *teratoasthenozoospermia* is often used to describe these associated abnormalities. When such abnormalities are associated with reduced numbers of sperm in an ejaculate, the term *oligoteratoasthenozoospermia* may also be used!

It is now of value to consider the ways in which sperm may be prepared for morphological assessment.

Light microscopy

Wet preparation

This is a quick but unreliable method of assessing sperm morphology and certainly must not be used by the inexperienced technician. A drop of undiluted semen is put onto a clean glass slide on top of which is placed a coverslip. These motile sperm are then examined and the percentage of abnormal sperm present estimated. As many of the sperm are motile, their morphology is often hard to define. It is also difficult in an unstained specimen to identify the origins of particulate matter and cellular debris that may be present in these men. Nuclear detail is entirely absent and there is no way by which a premalignant cell can be identified. However, such an assessment may be used on an interim report should it be necessary.

Stained preparation

A drop of well mixed undiluted semen is placed on one end of a clean glass slide and a smear is made in exactly the same way as for a blood film. The smear is then air dried and fixed. The stains used vary from laboratory to laboratory and will also depend on the availability of each stain. In most laboratories, one of three stains is used most frequently: these are haematoxylin and eosin (Table 9.1), Papanicalaou (Table 9.2) or May Grunwald Giemsa (Table 9.3). All the stains used in these protocols are available commercially.

Haematoxylin and eosin

This simple stain is available in all laboratories and for the most part is adequate for staining spermatozoa (Plate 9.1). The stain consists of Harris' haematoxylin and a 0.5% solution of eosin. The method has the advantage of speed and simplicity.

Table 9.1. The method of staining spermatozoa with Haematoxylin and Eosin (Bancroft & Cook, 1984)

1. Air dry smear of semen
2. Fix in methanol
3. Wash well with water
4. Immerse in freshly filtered Harris's Haematoxylin for 1 minute
5. Wash in water
6. Immerse in acid–alcohol (1% HCl in 70% alcohol) for 2–3 minutes
7. Wash in water
8. Dip into a 2% sodium bicarbonate solution for 10–20 seconds
9. Wash well in water
10. Stain with an aqueous 0.5% solution of Eosin for 20 seconds
11. Wash in water
12. Clear and mount

Table 9.2. A modification of the Papanicolaou stain used by the Department of Pathology, City Hospital, Nottingham. It is a simplification of the original Papanicolaou stain and produces good morphological detail in sperm

Modified Papanicolaou Stain

The semen is spread thinly on clean glass slide and air dried. The slide is then immersed for fixed times in the following solutions:

1.	Fix Methanol	20 minutes
2.	70% Alcohol	1 minute
3.	Distilled water	1 minute
4.	Harris's Haemotoxylin	3 seconds
5.	Running tap water	1 minute
6.	1.5% Acid–alcohol solution	15 seconds
7.	Running tap water	3 minutes
8.	70% alcohol	1 minute
9.	Absolute alcohol	1 minute
10.	Orange G	45 seconds
11.	Absolute alcohol	1 minute
12.	Absolute alcohol	1 minute
13.	Papanicolaou EA 50	1.5 minutes
14.	Absolute alcohol × 3 (wash)	
15.	Xylene clear in two separate aliquots of Xylene	
16.	Mount using 'DPX'	

Table 9.3. The protocol for staining spermatozoa using the May Grunwald Giemsa method

---

Air Dry

A smear of semen is made on a glass slide and then air dried. The slide is then immersed in the following solutions:

1.	Methanol	5 minutes
2.	May Grunwald Giemsa	5 minutes
3.	May Grunwald/Sorenson's Buffer	10 minutes
4.	Giemas/Sorenson's Buffer	10 minutes
	(May Grunwald 100 ml, Sorenson's Buffer 400 ml)	
5.	Aceton (quick wash)	
6.	Aceton–Xylene (equal volumes) quick wash	
7.	Clean in 2 aliquots of Zylene	
8.	Mount with DPX	

Papanicalaou

This stain requires a complex protocol but produces excellent cytological and in particular nuclear detail (Fig. 9.1). It is probably the best stain of all for spermatozoa and is particularly useful in demonstrating immature cells.

May Grunwald Giemsa

This staining protocol also gives good results but may not be so freely available within a pathology department as is the Papanicalaou Stain which is routinely used by any laboratory performing diagnostic cytology. However good cytological detail is obtained using Giemsa. The nucleii and the tails of the spermatozoa stain dark blue. The results are well worth the effort in using this particular staining technique (Fig. 9.1).

The choice of stain, however, depends mostly on the method one is most familiar with and which is almost readily available in your particular laboratory. Many other methods may also be used provided that they reliably stain the head, midpiece and also the tail of every spermatozoa. If one is in a situation where staining techniques are, for some reason, impossible to carry out, an expensive but otherwise satisfactory alternative is to use 'Testsimplets®'. These are glass slides manufactured by Boehringer Corporation (London) Ltd. A drop of semen is placed on a pre-stained slide and after 15 minutes is examined under a coverslip. If the coverslip is sealed, the stain retains its colour for up to 5 days. However, few pathology departments would have need of such a kit but this method may be of value to General Practitioners without access to a laboratory.

Morphological abnormalities that may be present in sperm

The well known pleomorphism of spermatozoa makes their assessment into 'normal' and 'abnormal' forms very difficult indeed. However, groups of well described abnormalities may be present in semen that can involve the head or the tail and on occasions, all parts of the sperm.

Head abnormalities

The size of sperm heads vary but if there is a marked reduction or an obvious increase in head size, these sperm must be deemed to be abnormal. The presence of vacuoles within the head must also be noted. The head may also be tapering or pyriform (Plate 9.2). Such head shapes are said to occur more frequently in the semen of infertile men with a varicocoele (MacLeod, 1965) and their presence in semen samples should be reported. Some sperm also show a dense head staining with a reduced or absent acrosome and as such may not be fertile. Amorphous, illshaped heads also occur in semen and are likely to be infertile. Conjoined sperm may also be found in increased numbers in infertile semen and these conjoined sperm also frequently show other abnormalities, particularly of their heads.

Tail abnormalities

Tail defects also frequently occur amongst sperm from infertile patients. The presence of sperm with coiled tails are a particularly bad prognostic sign in infertile semen but one must remember that tail abnormalities can easily be induced during a semen analysis particularly if the semen has been diluted. Care must therefore be taken to exclude artefact before reporting these abnormalities. Other tail abnormalities include eccentrically inserted tails (which are often wrongly called broken necks) and hair-pin deformities. Short stubby tails may also occur as can duplicate or even triplicate tails (Plate 9.3). Midpiece defects particularly involving the mitochondrial helix may also be found.

Immature sperm are characterized by the presence of a structure known as a cytoplasmic droplet (Fig. 9.1). This droplet may represent

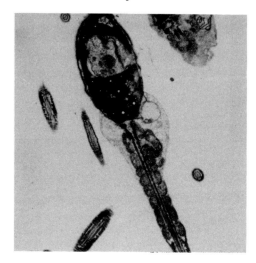

Fig. 9.1. Cytoplasmic droplets on a spermatozoan. Best demonstrated using electron microscopy.

part of the cytoplasm of the Sertoli cell from whence this sperm recently came.

Described above are some of the more common abnormalities that may be seen among a population of sperm in a sample of semen.

Counting abnormal sperm in a semen specimen

In order that the abnormal sperm are correctly identified, it is very important that they are examined at a sufficiently high magnification. Also, in order that the incidence of these abnormalities is statistically meaningful, a large enough number of sperm must be examined. It is therefore suggested that the stained smear be examined at a magnification of at least × 1000 and this means that an oil immersion must be used with a correctly adjusted bright field illumination. A total of at least 100 spermatozoa must be examined and the abnormalities amongst these counted at the same time. If either 100 or 200 sperm are examined, the percentage incidence of each of the abnormalities is then easy to calculate.

For practical purposes, spermatozoa are counted using a simple manual cell counter. As each abnormal sperm is encountered, the type of abnormality is charted. The total number of abnormal sperm seen is then expressed on the report as a percentage. If one abnormality

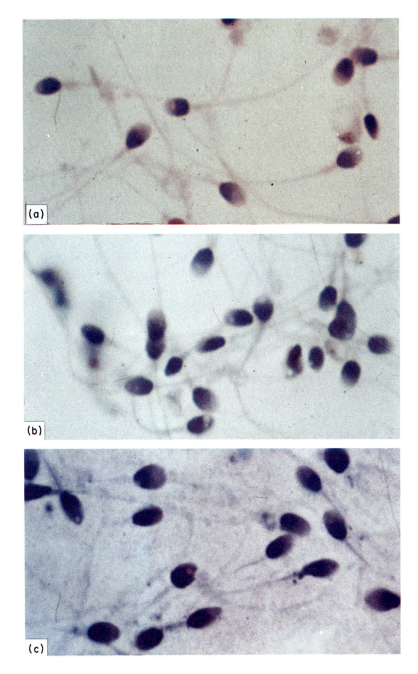

Plate 9.1. Normal sperm stained with (a) haematoxylin and eosin; (b) the Papanicolaou stain; and (c) May Grunwald Giemsa stain.

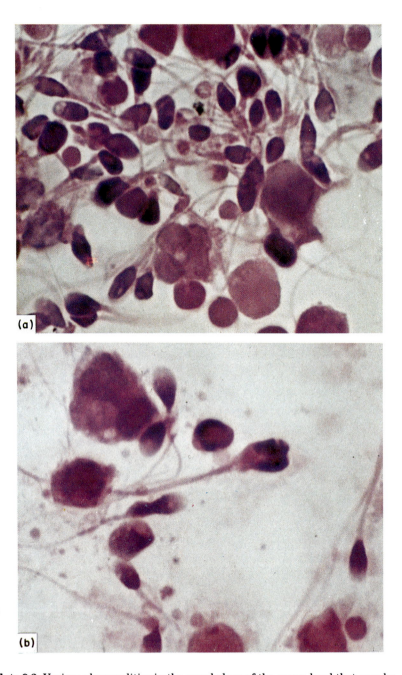

Plate 9.2. Various abnormalities in the morphology of the sperm head that may be seen in the examination of a semen specimen. These abnormalities include (a) round heads, amorphous heads, tapered heads and heads showing vacuolation and abnormalities of the chromatin. The lower photograph (b) shows a double-headed sperm.

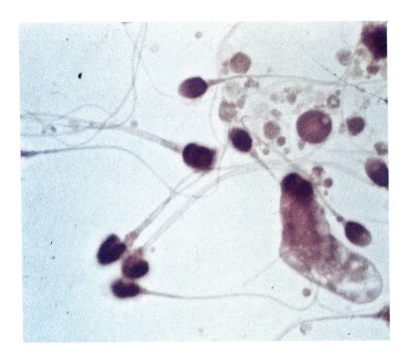

Plate 9.3. Abnormalities in the necks and tails of spermatozoa that can be found during the examination of semen. The top of the photo-micrograph shows sperm with abnormal mid-pieces. The lower area of the photo-micrograph shows spermatozoa with double tails.

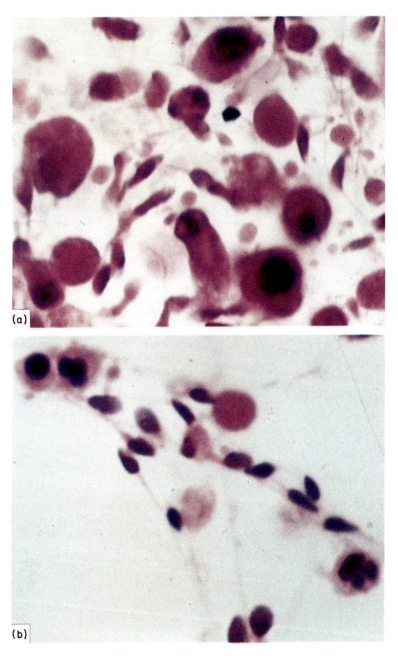

Plate 9.4. Photomicrographs of seminal fluid containing excess numbers of (a) germinal cells; and (b) leucocytes (stained with haematoxylin and eosin).

presents more than 20% of the total abnormalities, then this fact should certainly be indicated on the report. For more accurate reporting, especially that associated with any research project, the percentage incidence of each abnormality is detailed on a much more complicated report (WHO, 1980), a variant of which is used by the authors (Table 9.4).

Table 9.4. A method of reporting the various abnormalities of sperm morphology that may be seen in a semen specimen (WHO, 1980)

Cell Abnormality	%age
Normal spermatozoa	
Large oval head	
Small oval head	
Tapering head	
Pyriform head	
Amorphous head	
Double head	
Midpiece defects	
Double tails	
Coiled tails	
Short tails	
Cytoplasmic droplets	
Immature germ cells	
White blood cells	

White blood cells

The white blood cell is present in small numbers in normal semen but presence in semen in large numbers indicates inflammation (Plate 9.4). This problem will be discussed in more detail in the next section. The numbers of white cells must be counted on the stained smear as part of the morphological assessment of semen. The white cells should be expressed as the number per 100 spermatozoa. As the number of sperm per ml is already known, a rough estimate of the number of white blood cells present in 1 ml of semen may be calculated.

Other cellular components of semen

Although spermatozoa are by far the most numerous of the cells contained in semen, epithelial cells, red and white cells and even protozoa may also be present.

Epithelial cells

These arise from the lining of the genital tract and are always present in semen. They are occasionally present in excess in semen from men with urethritis. Even when they are present in large numbers, they have never been associated with the presence of any pathology. It may be of value to report them if they are present in large numbers.

Red blood cells

These cells are not usually present in semen. If blood is present in any amount, it colours semen red. If red cells are present in semen, it may be a manifestation of infection or possibly of malignant disease within the genital tract. The presence of red cells in semen and an approximate estimate of their concentration *must* be included on the report.

Germinal cells

These represent preformed sperm and are very often present in semen (Plate 9.4). Germinal cells are deemed usual in normal semen. However, the exact numbers of these immature cells that constitute an abnormality has not been determined. Nevertheless, their presence in a semen sample should be reported. They can only reliably be identified in a stained smear. Germinal cells are best expressed as cells per 100 spermatozoa and should be counted alongside the sperm during the assessment of sperm morphology. If the number of germinal cells per 100 spermatozoa is known then their approximate numbers per ml can also be calculated.

Lymphocytes

These round white cells may also be present in semen and may be difficult to distinguish from 'round' germinal cells. Their numbers are also best expressed as cells per 100 spermatozoa.

Protozoa and bacteria

The obvious presence of protozoa or bacteria in semen clearly indicates an infection. The most common protozoan is *Trichomas* which inhabits the anterior urethra but which rarely infects the posterior genital tract. In the same way, a *Candida* species may also contaminate semen. Visible bacteria in semen are also usually only contaminants: examples of these organisms are *Staphylococcus epidermidis* and *Streptococcus viridans*. Such findings must be indicated on the report. If visible bacteria are present especially in association with an excess of white cells, the semen sample should be sent for microbiological culture.

Particulate matter that may be present in semen

The particulate matter found in semen is usually obvious at the initial examination. Crystals of endogenous substances such as spermine may be present but one may also see crystals of exogenous substances such as talcum powder and the spermicidal powders from the inside of a contraceptive sheath (Fig. 9.2). It is not uncommon to see prostatic calculii in semen. Such particles need not be included on a report unless they are present in excess or unless they are clearly substances, such as spermicidal agents, that will interfere with the activity of sperm.

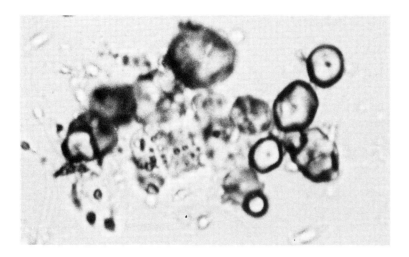

Fig. 9.2. Crystals that can be seen during the routine microscopy of semen. These substances commonly include talcum powder, spermicidal powder from a condom and spermine crystals. An example of talc crystals in semen is given above.

Electron microscopy of sperm

Electron microscopy has been used extensively in the examination of mammalian sperm and has considerably aided diagnosis in a number of different types of male infertility. However, electron microscopy is expensive and time-consuming and therefore cannot, and indeed should not, be applied to every semen specimen undergoing routine analysis. However for specific abnormalities, the electron microscope is very valuable indeed and it may be the only way in which a particular abnormality may be diagnosed.

Sperm may be evaluated using either scanning electron microscopy (SEM) or sperm may be examined after sectioning in the technique known as transmission electron microscopy (TEM).

Scanning electron microscopy (SEM)

This technique allows examination of the outer coverings of the spermatozoa and provides a good view of a spermatozoon as a whole. Indeed it was using this technique that much of the knowledge concerning the general shape and appearances of the cell membrane of the sperm was first acquired. It is beyond the scope of this book to describe in detail the way in which sperm are prepared for scanning electron microscopy and the technique varies considerably from laboratory to laboratory. A commonly used method is that freshly ejaculated sperm are removed from liquified semen, washed several times in sucrose citrate, fixed in buffered glutaraldehyde, washed again in buffered sucrose and then dehydrated in alcohol. The sperm are then placed on a clean coverslip and air dried. It is however very easy in any technique used to prepare sperm for SEM to cause artefactual damage.

Diagnostically, scanning electron microscopy demonstrates clearly all the gross abnormalities of sperm that may be associated with infertility. Abnormalities of the sperm heads are particularly vividly demonstrated using this technique. However all these abnormalities can usually be identified using light microscopy, provided care is taken to stain and examine the sperm properly. It is the authors' belief that scanning electron microscopy has little to offer in the routine examination of infertile semen.

Transmission electron microscopy (TEM)

If the spermatozoa are pelleted, fixed and sectioned and then viewed electron microscopically, many abnormalities most particularly of the axoneme may be demonstrated which otherwise would go unrecognized.

This technique known as transmission electron microscopy (TEM) is indeed of use when applied to sperm in the diagnosis of male infertility. However, the value of TEM is for the most part in the diagnosis of disorders of the axoneme (contractile elements of the sperm) and therefore is usually only of value when applied to sperm showing abnormalities or absence of movement.

The method of preparation of spermatozoa for TEM again varies considerably between laboratories but basically sperm are first extracted from freshly ejaculated liquified semen and fixed with glutaraldehyde. After staining with osmium tetroxide and embedding in agar, the block is cut on an ultramicrotome to provide 0.5 μm sections which are mounted and examined.

A number of different anomalies may be seen (Fig. 9.3). One of the most common is the absence of the dynein arms. These structures contain the energy source for the contractile elements without which the tail cannot move. Absence of the nexin links and also the radial links may also be found. Absence of the central 2 contractile elements producing the so-called '9+0' phenomenon results in total immobilization of the sperm. This abnormality may be associated with severe chest disease in the patient when it is known clinically as Kartageners Syndrome or the Immotile Cilia Syndrome (Eliasson *et al.*, 1977). One other not infrequent cause of sperm immotility is an absence or abnormality of the proximal centriole. Thus TEM can be very valuable in diagnosing 'internal' disorders of sperm morphology but which frequently involve the contractile elements of the sperm. Thus TEM is really only of value in the investigation of disorders of sperm movement.

One aspect of the use of electron microscopy in relation to sperm morphology that must not be forgotten is the very great possibility of what is known as sampling error. During the examination of say 5 or 6 sections, it may only be possible to visualize 20–30 sperm tails. Thus if these sperm have formed part of an ejaculate containing 30 million sperm, one has only examined 0.000001% of the sperm in that ejaculate, and thus the TEM findings might not be truly representative of the ejaculate as a whole. There is, however, little one can do about this problem except to be aware of this as a possible source of error in the ultrastructural evaluation of a semen sample.

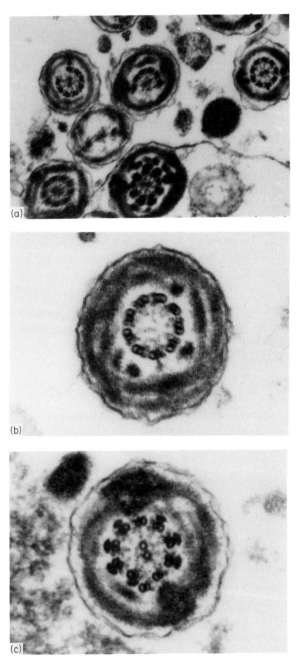

Fig. 9.3. Transmission electron micrographs showing a variety of different abnormalities in the axoneme of sperm tails. These include (a) a variety of diferent abnormalities of the microtubules; (b) the '9+0' abnormality; and (c) lack of dynein arms.

References

Bancroft, J. D. & Cook, H. C. (1984) *Manual of Histological Techniques*. Churchill Livingstone, Edinburgh.

Eliasson, R., Mossberg, B., Camner, P. & Afzelius, B. A. (1977) The Immotile Cilia Syndrome. A congenital ciliary abnormality as an aetiologic factor in chronic airway infections and male infertility. *New England Journal of Medicine* **297**, 1–6.

MacLeod, J. (1965) Seminal cytology in the presence of varicocoele. *Fertility and Sterility* **16**, 735–57.

WHO Special Programme of Research, Development and Research Training in Human Reproduction. (1980) *Laboratory Manual for the Examination of Human Semen and Semen-Cervical Mucus Interaction*, p. 25–7. Press Concern, Singapore.

10

Useful Biochemical Tests

Human seminal plasma is a highly complex mixture of many different biochemical substances which include proteins, amines, carbohydrates, lipids and electrolytes. A few are specific to certain parts of the genital tract and a demonstration of their presence or absence in semen can be of great value diagnostically (Table 10.1). The compounds in semen that are at present useful in diagnosis are relatively few, but it is likely that this aspect of semen analysis will have increasing importance. Some of the substances in semen which may one day be of value diagnostically will also be discussed in this section.

Table 10.1. Biochemical changes that may be seen in the semen of men with a variety of different causes of infertility

Genital tract lesion causing infertility	Sperm concentration	pH of semen	Seminal volume	Seminal fructose	Seminal acid phosphatase/ citrate
Bilateral epididiymal obstruction	Azoospermia	Normal	Normal	Normal	Normal
Congenital absence of vasa deferentia	Azoospermia	Normal, or reduced	Reduced	Absent	Raised
Ejaculatory duct obstructions	Azoospermia	Normal, or reduced	Reduced	Absent	Raised
Polyzoospermia	Raised ($>350 \times 10^6$)	Normal	Normal	Reduced	Normal

Fructose

Fructose is present in large quantities in semen and is the main energy source for the sperm (Mann & Rottenberg, 1966). It is produced by the seminal vesicles. A congenital absence of the seminal vesicles (Amelar & Hotchkiss, 1963) — a not uncommon anomaly often associated with

76

absence of both vasa deferentia — or obliteration of seminal vesicular secretions by infection, will result in a reduction in the amount of fructose in semen (Eliasson, 1971). Impairment of seminal vesicular secretion will result in reduced fructose concentrations in semen and motility of the sperm may be reduced. As the seminal vesicles contribute more than half of the total volume of semen, absence of the seminal vesicular secretions will reduce the seminal volume. Thus the measurement of fructose concentration in men with low volume ejaculates may be of great value diagnostically (Phadke *et al.*, 1973). When the seminal vesicular contributions are absent, the substances present in the prostatic contribution to semen will thus be in an increased concentration in semen.

Another situation where fructose estimations are helpful are in men with polyzoospermia and low motility (Amelar *et al.*, 1979). Occasionally in men with very high sperm concentrations (more than 350 million sperm per ml), the sperm are immotile due to a relative deficiency of fructose. If this semen picture is present, the diagnosis may be confirmed by finding very low concentrations or even an absence of fructose in the semen.

Fructose is measured in most chemical pathology departments — a common method used in the resorcinol test of Seliwanoff. The concentration of fructose in semen ranges from 3.5–28 mmol/l. It must be remembered that as the semen sample ages, the fructose level will fall due to the utilization of fructose by the spermatozoa. The more sperm that are present in the ejaculate, the greater the fall in fructose concentration.

Acid phosphatase

Acid phosphatase is secreted into the semen by the prostate gland and is therefore a useful marker of prostatic function. It is a very stable enzyme and for this reason it is used by forensic laboratories as a test for the presence of semen. It may also be used as a test for the presence of a prostatic contribution in an ejaculate.

Acid phosphatase is measured by all clinical chemistry departments. The method used is one involving the action of this enzyme on a substrate. Acid phosphatase is found in semen in concentrations of 88–979 iu/100 ml.

Citric acid

Citric acid is also present in prostatic fluid and may also be used as a marker of prostatic secretion. It is measured spectrophotometrically but its assay is less often used than that of acid phosphatase and it is thus less easy to obtain assays for citric acid than for acid phosphatase. Citric acid is present in semen at concentrations of 20–39 mmol.

Zinc

Much attention has been paid recently to zinc in semen (Eliasson & Lindholmer, 1971). Zinc is secreted by the prostate and stabilizes seminal proteins. Its role in male infertility remains uncertain. It can also be used as a prostatic marker. It is measured by automated spectrophotometry and is present in semen in concentrations of 25–424 µg/ml.

Other compounds present in semen which may have diagnostic value in the future

Prostaglandins

Prostaglandins and in particular PGF_2 play an important role in contracting smooth muscle. All the prostaglandins are present in quite high concentrations in semen and are secreted by the seminal vesicles (Eliasson, 1959). It has been suggested that prostaglandins stimulate contraction of the urethral smooth muscle during ejaculation and may aid sperm transport in the female. They may also enhance sperm penetration of cervical mucus. The concentration of prostaglandins in semen may be reduced in infertile men but the mechanism of this reduction is not understood. When the role of prostaglandins in infertility is clarified, measurement of seminal fluid prostaglandins may have diagnostic value.

LDH-C_4

An enzyme known as LDH-C_4 is specific to sperm. It may be released into semen when sperm die and disintegrate (Gavella *et al.*, 1982). Assay of this enzyme may one day also prove useful in determining whether sperm are not being released into the genital tract or whether poor survival is the problem. The use of this assay in seminology and its use diagnostically is still being evaluated.

Transferrin

Transferrin is produced and released into the testicular component of the semen by the Sertoli cells. It may therefore be a useful marker for Sertoli cell function. Transferrin is present in relatively low concentrations in semen and the normal assays used to measure transferrin in blood are not sensitive enough. Whether, using specially developed radioimmunoassays (Holmes *et al.*, 1982), the measurement of seminal transferrin will prove to be useful diagnostically, remains to be seen.

Inhibin

Inhibin is the name given to a substance or group of substances produced by the Sertoli cells. The main action of inhibin is to feedback onto the pituitary and suppress follicle stimulating hormone secretion. However, inhibin appears to be secreted into the seminal fluid and may act as a Sertoli cell marker. The assay of inhibin is very laborious and difficult (Hudson *et al.*, 1979). Inhibin may prove a very valuable diagnostic marker in the future, provided the problems with its measurement are resolved.

It should now be clear that biochemistry has an important part to play in the evaluation of a semen sample. It is likely that in the future this role will be considerably increased and that semen analysis will extend far beyond the microscope and the counting of sperm.

References

Amelar, R. D. & Hotchkiss, R. S. (1963) Congenital aplasia of the epididymes and vasa deferentia: Effects on semen. *Fertility and Sterility* 14, 44–8.

Amelar, R. D., Dubin, L., Quigley, M. M. & Schoenfeld, C. (1979) Successful management of infertility due to polyzoospermia. *Fertility and Sterility* 31, 521–4.

Eliasson, R. (1959) Studies on prostaglandin occurrence, formation and biological action. *Acta Physiologica Scandinavica* 46 (Suppl. 158), 1–73.

Eliasson, R. (1971) Standards for the investigation of human semen. *Andrologie* 3, 49–64.

Eliasson, R. & Lindholmer, C. (1971) Zinc in human seminal plasma. *Andrologie* 3, 147–53.

Gavella, M., Cvitkovic, P. & Skrabalo, Z. (1982) Seminal plasma isoenzyme LDHX in infertile men. *Andrologie* 14, 104–9.

Holmes, S. D., Lipshultz, L. I. & Smith, R. G. (1982) Transferrin and gonadal dysfunction in man. *Fertility and Sterility* **38**, 600–4.

Hudson, B., Baker, H. W. G., Eddie, L. W., Higginson, R. E., Burger, H. G., de Kretser, D. M., Dobbs, M. & Lee, V. W. K. (1979) Bioassays for inhibin: A critical review. *Journal of Reproduction and Fertility* (Suppl. 26), 17–29.

Mann, T. and Rottenberg, D. A. (1966) The carbohydrate of human semen. *Journal of Endocrinology* **34**, 257–64.

Phadke, A. M., Samant, N. R. & Deval, S. P. (1973) Significance of seminal fructose studies in male infertility. *Fertility and Sterility* **24**, 894–903.

11

Problem of Immotile Sperm

The scientific staff involved in the performance of semen analyses can, on many occasions, be of great help to the clinician by applying certain tests to sperm which are outside the normal routine of a semen analysis and which may not even have been requested by the clinician. This is nowhere better illustrated than in the investigation of semen containing numerous immotile sperm. In this section, it is proposed to discuss the ways in which semen analysis staff may aid in the diagnosis of asthenozoospermia and provide the clinician not only with the finding of immotile sperm but also with its cause.

Let us first suppose that the semen under investigation has been provided by the male partner of an infertile couple and only 10% of the sperm are showing any movement. The possible reasons for this finding are outlined below.

Artefact

Even very minor contamination of semen by a wide variety of substances may be sufficient to immobilize and kill spermatozoa. Containers contaminated with water, soap or detergent for example, may cause artefactual asthenozoospermia. Likewise, if semen comes into contact with rubber as would happen if the container had a rubber lined lid, sperm immotility will result. It is therefore important that the clinician is made aware of this and should a semen sample appear in the laboratory in any container other than the standard one, this fact must be made clear on the report.

If the semen specimen is old or has been subjected to cold, asthenozoospermia may result. It is the responsibility of the clinician to instruct the patient clearly about the collection of the semen and its transport to the laboratory. However, semen can be left in a cold place after its delivery to the laboratory and as sperm are easily damaged by temperatures of less than 20°C, artefactual immobilization of sperm can occur after the specimen has arrived at the laboratory. Placing the semen sample in an incubator for 30 minutes results in a return of motility and thus will prove that the immotility was indeed due to cold.

Despite instructions to the contrary, there are still patients who produce specimens in a condom. Many condoms contain spermicidal powder and even in the absence of such a powder, the volatile hydrocarbons within the interslices of the rubber are very toxic to sperm. The presence of large numbers of the characteristic crystals of the spermicidal agent make this diagnosis very easy. Any possibility of the production of the semen specimen into a condom must be included on the report.

Deficiency of fructose

Fructose is an important source of energy for movement by the sperm and thus any deficiency of fructose in seminal fluid may result in asthenozoospermia. Fructose is produced by the seminal vesicles and is present in their secretions. Failure of development of the seminal vesicles or damage to their secretions may result in a reduction in the concentration of fructose in semen and an associated asthenozoospermia. As the seminal vesicles supply more than half of the total ejaculatory volume, this diagnosis would be supported by a semen sample of low volume. A simple test for this phenomenon is to take an aliquot of this semen and add an isotonic sugar solution to it. The simplest isotonic sugar solution to use is Baker's buffer (Rose *et al.*, 1976). This is non-toxic to sperm and contains 3% glucose (Table 11.1). If the asthenozoospermia is due to fructose deficiency, addition of Baker's buffer should produce an immediate resumption of sperm motility. An equal volume of Baker's buffer (warm — not straight out of the fridge!) is added to a small aliquot of semen on a glass slide and

Table 11.1. The formulation of Baker's buffer

Glucose	3.0 g
$Na_2H\,PO_4 \cdot 7H_2O$	0.46 g
or	
$Na_2H\,PO_4 \cdot 12H_2O$	0.6 g
NaCl	0.2 g
$KH_2\,PO_4$	0.01 g
Distilled water up to 100 ml	

the two are gently mixed. The change in motility is diagnostic of fructose deficiency. A larger aliquot of semen may now be sent to the clinical chemistry department for assay of fructose. However a second sample of semen may be needed for the estimation of fructose as at least 1 ml of fluid is required for this assay. This simple test is most helpful diagnostically for the clinician in identifying disorders of the seminal vesicles.

Another cause of fructose deficiency which is less commonly seen is that due to polyzoospermia (Amelar *et al.*, 1979). In this situation, high concentrations of sperm (usually in excess of 350 million/ml) cause too rapid utilization of fructose and consequently loss of motility. Addition of Baker's buffer will also make the diagnosis here too. The absence of response to Baker's buffer excludes fructose deficiency and makes the measurement of the seminal fructose unnecessary.

Infection

The presence of infection, a situation often manifested by the presence of excess white cells and even visible bacteria can also cause sperm immotility. Findings such as these indicate the need for bacterial culture of the semen. If these abnormalities are seen during a semen analysis, it is of great help if an aliquot of the semen sample is sent for culture straight away. This may cut out the need for a further semen sample and will considerably speed up diagnosis.

Defects of the axoneme

As has already been described previously, poorly motile or immotile sperm may be the result of abnormalities of the axoneme. In some laboratories it may be possible to consider transmission electron microscopy of semen in these circumstances. It must be remembered however that all other causes of immotility must be excluded before this expensive and time-consuming investigation is undertaken. Also transmission electron microscopy must be performed using a very fresh sample of semen.

In this short section, a number of ways are described in which the laboratory may diagnostically aid the clinician. This type of help speeds up diagnosis and thus treatment of the infertile patient.

References

Amelar, R. D., Dubin, L., Quigley, M. M. & Schonfeld, C. (1979) Successful management of infertility due to polyzoospermia. *Fertility and Sterility* **31,** 521–4.

Rose, N. R., Hjort, T., Rumke, P., Harper, M. J. K. & Vyazov, O. (1976) Techniques for the detection of iso- and auto-antibodies to human spermatozoa. *Clinical and Experimental Immunology* **23,** 175–99.

12

Pyospermia and the Microbiology of Semen

Genital tract infection can, on occasions, be a cause of infertility in men. One of the ways in which these infections may become manifest is by the presence of excessive numbers of white blood cells in semen (Fig. 12.1). Increased numbers of white cells in semen is known as *pyospermia*. Many infective disorders of the genital tract are associated with symptoms and these may include testicular or epididymal pain as well as discomfort or pain on passing urine, pain on ejaculation or even the presence of blood in the semen. Blood stained semen is known as haematospermia. The presence of white blood cells lying together in aggregates is diagnostic of infection and any semen sample showing this phenomenon *must* be examined microbiologically. Thus a semen sample obtained from a patient with symptoms suggestive of

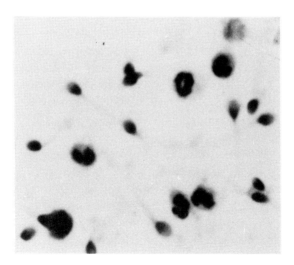

Fig. 12.1. A smear of semen showing a gross excess of white blood cells.

the presence of a genital tract infection should be examined microbiologically and the presence or absence of pyospermia should be
ascertained in all semen samples sent for analysis.

Increased numbers of white blood cells in semen generally indicates the presence of infection but may also be the result of prostatic
abnormalities. For this reason, pyospermia may be more commonly
seen in older men. However, excess numbers of white cells in semen
always indicates the need for microbiological investigation. A semen
sample found to show pyospermia must therefore always be sent for
culture.

Sites of infection that may produce pyospermia

There are three main sites for infection in the male genital tract. These
are the epididymis, the seminal vesicles and the prostate. The urethra
together with the urethra and bulbo-urethral glands may also be a site
of infection and thus of white cell production.

The split ejaculate

The exact site of production of the white cells can, if desired, by determined by the production of a 'split' ejaculate. During emission and
ejaculation, the secretions of the accessory glands together with the
testicular contribution, are discharged into the posterior urethra and
thus into the ejaculate in a predetermined sequence. The first part of
the ejaculate to be propelled out of the urethra is made up of the
testicular component of the semen followed by the secretions of the
prostate. Lastly the secretions of the seminal vesicles are expelled. It is
therefore possible for a patient to collect the semen in 'aliquots' as it
emerges from the urethra at ejaculation. This manoeuvre allows one to
examine each 'fraction' of the semen separately and also to investigate
the site of production of numerous substances in semen. It also allows
one to identify the site of an infection.

It is often possible for men to split the ejaculate into 3 or even as
many as 6 separate fractions (Eliasson & Lindholmer, 1976). The
patients are provided with a series of semen pots which are taped together (Fig. 12.2). It is also easy for the patient to ejaculate into small
trays which have been divided into a total of 6 separate boxes. The
divided specimens of semen are then analysed individually. The
technique of split ejaculate production can be applied to many aspects

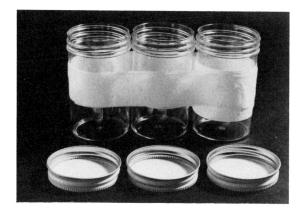

Fig. 12.2. Pots taped together for use in obtaining a split ejaculate.

of andrology. It has even been used to trace the site of entry of drugs and toxins into the seminal fluid.

Expressed prostatic secretion

As the prostate is an important site of infection, another method for detecting infection in the prostate is by used *expressed prostatic secretion*. Small amounts of fluid containing urine, seminal fluid and prostatic fluid can be obtained by prostatic massage per rectum. These samples are sent to the laboratory for cytological and bacteriological assessment.

The estimation of the number of white blood cells in a semen sample

The number of white blood cells present in semen is best reported as the number present either in a millilitre of semen or in the whole ejaculate. Some centres however persist in simply describing the number of white cells present per high power field.

Methods used to estimate white cell numbers in semen

Neubauer Counting Chamber

With experience it will become possible to perform a white cell count in semen using this counting chamber which, after all, was one of the functions for which it was designed. If the white cell count is performed using the improved Neubauer Counting Chamber, white cell diluting fluid must be used. Despite the staining that the white cell diluting fluid imparts to the cells, it is still extremely easy to mistake a germinal cell for a white cell and vice versa. For this reason, this method is not recommended for use by the inexperienced.

Stained smears

The white cell content of semen is best estimated using stained smears and can be performed at the same time as the assessment of the morphology. The smears can be stained using any of the three stains: haematoxylin and eosin, Papanicolaou or May Grunwald Giemsa (see Chapter 9).

Testsimplets

In situations where access to a laboratory and cytological stains may be difficult, special pre-stained slides known as 'Testsimplets' (Boehringer, Mannheim, W Germany) may be used. These have already been described in relation to the assessment of sperm morphology (see Chapter 9) and are also very good for estimating white cell numbers of semen.

Ways of counting white cells in semen

Number of white cells per high power field (hpf)

Many laboratories feel that it is quite adequate to report the white cell content of semen as the numbers of white cells present per high power field. As the magnification used should be of the order of $\times 400$ and the thickness of the semen smear (if made by a practiced hand) is likely not to vary substantially in thickness, reasonably accurate estimations of white cell numbers in terms of concentration can be achieved. The presence of up to 5 white blood cells per high power field is generally deemed to be normal. The white cell content can be reported as the mean number of white cells per high power field after a minimum of 5 fields have been examined. The white blood cell concentration can also be described semi-quantitatively, the usual format for this method of reporting is:

5–20 WBC/hpf = 'increased'
20–40 WBC/hpf =   +
40+ WBC/hpf =   + +

Number of white cells per millilitre of semen

The number of white blood cells present in a semen sample is probably best reported as the concentration of white blood cells present either in 1 ml of semen or as the total number present in the ejaculate.

The concentration of white blood cells in semen can, of course, easily be estimated using the Improved Neubauer Counting Chamber. If, as is probably easier, a stained smear is used, the number of white blood cells alongside 100 spermatozoa are counted. Using duplicate fields, a mean value is obtained. Provided the sperm concentration is already known, the concentration of white blood cells per ml of semen can easily be calculated.

Number of white blood cells alongside 100 sperm = 2
Sperm concentration $= 100 \times 10^6$
White blood cell concentration $= 2 \times 10^6$

If the number of white blood cells present in an ejaculate is required, then this number must be multiplied by the ejaculatory volume.

It is generally agreed that while blood cell concentrations in excess of 5×10^6/ml or more (the same number in millions is the same as that described in relation to a high power field) must be deemed to be abnormal and likely to be indicative of the presence of infection. When split ejaculates are examined, the white blood cell count should be reported in relation to each fraction as this will indicate to the clinician the likely site of the infection.

How infection alters semen quality

Infection may alter semen quality in a number of different ways. Firstly, an infective process may damage the ductal system of the genital tract resulting in a partial or a totally obstructive lesion, a situation which most frequently involves the epididymis. Infection may also interfere with secretion from one of the accessory glands of the male genital tract: a good example of such a problem is where infection affects the seminal vesicles producing a reduction in the volume and quality of its secretions (Eliasson, 1971). The semen may as a consequence become reduced in volume and contain sperm that are reduced in motility because of a deficient concentration of fructose in the seminal plasma.

The presence of pus in semen appears to be associated with poor motility of the spermatozoa. How this phenomenon is brought about is not very clear. However there is evidence that *Escherichia coli* may produce an 'immobilization factor' for this has been isolated from *E. coli* filtrates (Paulson & Polakoski, 1977). In some cases, the bacteria may attack the sperm either by attaching itself to the sperm as may be the case in Chlamydial infections. Bacteria may also actually lyse the cell wall of the spermatozoa. It is clear however that both infection and the presence of a marked pyospermia can occur without there being any apparent detriment to semen quality.

Organisms that may be associated with pyospermia

Large numbers of different organisms have been described in semen in relation to pyospermia and infertility.

Escherichia Coli

Of all the organisms present in semen that can cause pyospermia, *E. coli* and other Gram-negative bacilli must be the most frequently identified. *E. coli* is often found in semen in patients with a history of an *E. coli* urinary infection and this organism appears to colonize the prostate. It may also induce the production of surface specific IgA and its presence may be detected by finding such an immunoglobulin in the semen or prostatic fluid (Shortcliffe *et al.*, 1981). *E. coli* is also known to induce sperm agglutination (Teague *et al.*, 1971). The finding of clumped sperm in a patient with pyospermia would very strongly suggest the presence of *E. coli*.

Enterococci

Organisms such as *Streptococcus faecalis* may also occasionally be found in association with pyospermia. However, great care must be taken not to assume that the presence of an organism in semen is necessarily the cause of the pyospermia. *Enterococci* are present in the urethra of many patients and for the most part may simply be a contaminant.

Staphylococci

Staphylococci, especially *Staphylococcus epidermidis*, is frequently present in the urethra and only very rarely have any pathological sigificance in the production of pyospermia. Here again, care must be taken not to assume that an organism that may be cultured in semen is the cause of the patient's infertility.

Neisseria gonorrhoeae

For the most part, gonorrhoeae in men produces severe symptoms and is thus easy to diagnose. For this reason it will only rarely present as simple infertility and pyospermia. As in other fluids however, *Neisseria gonorrhoeae* can be seen in semen as Gram-negative intracellular *diplococci* and its presence should always be sought in men with pyospermia.

Myocabacterium Tuberculosis

Tuberculosis is a rare cause of male infertility in Britain today but it can still present as a form of infertility which may be associated with pyospermia. However, it must be remembered that severe tuberculosis can be present in the absence of any pus in the semen and where its presence may only be manifest by the presence of red blood cells. Tuberculosis usually causes a variety of different obstructive lesions and thus the patient with this infection is frequently azoospermic (Hanley, 1955). Culture of semen for the possible presence of acid fast bacilli must be considered in a patient with azoospermia, pyospermia and in particular haematospermia.

Mycoplasmas

Trachomatis mycoplasma, now better known as *Ureaplasma urealyticum*, will colonize the male reproductive tract as will *Mycoplasma hominis*. Although there is no doubt that these organisms can be cultured from semen and may invade the prostate (Taylor-Robinson *et al.*, 1977), it is far less certain whether they are in fact a cause of infertility. However, there is suggestion that treatment of infertile patients shown to have *T. mycoplasma* in their semen with an appropriate antibiotic did improve sperm motility and thus enhance fertility (Swenson *et al.*, 1979).

Chlamydia

Chlamydia trachomatis may occasionally be found in human semen
and is known to be a cause of epididymitis (Berger *et al.*, 1978). It
would appear that if this organism causes epididymal damage, then infertility will result. One must presume that elimination of this
organism from the genital tract will at least prevent the infertility be-
coming worse. The presence or absence of Chlamydial antibodies in the
patient's serum may aid diagnosis.

Trichomonas vaginalis

T. vaginalis is frequently found in the anterior urethra and thus may
be seen in samples of seminal fluid. There is, however, no evidence that
T. vaginalis is ever a cause of either pyospermia or of male infertility
although *T. Vaginalis* may interfere to some extent with sperm
motility (Tuttle *et al.*, 1977).

Candida Albicans

C. albicans may also be present in semen. It usually only colonizes
smegma and thus must be considered only to be a contaminant of
semen. It does not cause infertility.

Viruses

The role of viruses in infection of the male reproductive tract and in
the production of infertility is very uncertain. Cytomegalovirus has
been found to cause infection of the genital tract but it appeared to
have only a minor effect on the semen quality. Smallpox virus was
known in the past to produce obstructive azoospermia (Phadke *et al.*,
1973).

Genital herpes virus has frequently been isolated from semen and
although it is likely that the male genital tract can act as a source or
reservoir for herpes infection, there is little evidence that it has any
deleterious effect on testicular or epididymal function.

In the majority of patients with pyospermia, the sad fact is that no
causative organism can be found in semen to explain its presence.
However all samples of semen that are found to contain excessive
numbers of white cells must be subjected to microbiological
examination.

The microbiological examination of semen

The culture of organisms in seminal fluid can be difficult for several reasons. Firstly, semen has a high pH (7–8) which does not provide optimum cultural conditions. Secondly, it contains large amounts of lysozymes and also of zinc, both of which are powerfully antibacterial. Semen that is sent for bacteriological culture must be fresh. Bacteria easily die in semen due to the presence of these antibacterial substances. Thus the application of the semen to the agar as quickly as possible will yield a higher rate of positive cultures.

The first step in the microbiological examination of semen is to make a smear and perform a Gram stain. The presence of a predominant type of organism may aid decisions concerning methods of culture. Such stains may also detect the presence of contaminants such as *Candida albicans*. In general, however, the methods of culture used in the bacteriological assessment of semen are simple.

Usually only three media are commonly used in the culture of semen. Tissue culture may also occasionally be employed.

Blood agar

Blood agar innoculated with neat semen will be sufficient to identify most of the organisms that may be present in semen. These organisms include *E. coli*, the *Enterococci* and *Staphylococci*. If the blood agar is incubated both in air and also anaerobically in carbon dioxide, *N. Gonorrhoeae* will also be identified.

Chocolate agar or New York city medium

This medium if cultured anaerobically is especially useful for the identification of *N. Gonorrhoeae*. If this infection is suspected in a patient (and in particular if intracellular Gram-negative diplococci were seen on the Gram stain), semen must be innoculated onto this medium.

Cystine-lactose-electrolyte-deficient (CLED) medium

This is a particularly good medium for the identification of *E. coli* and many other gut organisms. However, many of these grow equally well on blood agar. This medium is excellent for any lactose fermenting organisms such as *Enterococci*.

Tissue culture

This must be used for the positive identification of *Chlamydia*. In most patients the presence of a chlamydial infection is usually determined by the presence of a chlamydial antibody in the patient's serum. These methods for microbiological culture of semen are outlined in Table 12.1.

Table 12.1. A summary of the media that are commonly used in the microbiological examination of semen, together with the organisms that such media will identify

Blood agar	*Staphylococci, Enterococci, E. coli* etc.
Chocolate agar or New York City medium	*N. gonorrhoeae*
Cystine lactose electrolyte deficient (CLED) medium	*E. coli* and many of the gut organisms. Lactose *jermenters*
Tissue culture	Chlamydial organisms

The microbiological examination of semen thus forms a very important part of a semen analysis. Initiative taken by the laboratory staff in organizing the bacteriological examination of semen based on the findings at a semen analysis will be most helpful to the clinician and provide a considerable saving in time for the patient in that the cause of his infertility may be determined that much more quickly.

References

Berger, R. E., Alexander, E. R., Monda, E. D., Ansell, J., McCormick, G. & Holmes, K. K. (1978) *Chlamydia trachomalis* as a cause of acute 'idiopathic' epididymitis. *New England Journal of Medicine* **298**, 301–4.

Eliasson, R. (1977) Standards for the investigation of human semen. *Andrologie* **3**, 49–64.

Eliasson, R. & Lindholmer, C. (1976) Functions of male accessory genital organs. In Hafez, E. S. E. (ed) *Human Semen and Fertility Regulation in Men*, pp. 44–50. Mosby, St. Louis.

Hanley, H. G. (1955) The surgery of male subfertility. *Annals of the Royal College of Surgeons.* **17**, 159–83.

Paulson, J. D. & Polakoski, K. J. (1977) Isolation of spermatozoal immobilisation factor from *Escherichia coli* filtrates. *Fertility and Sterility* **28**, 182–5.

Phadke, A. M., Samant, N. R. & Deval, S. D. (1973) Smallpox as an aetiological factor in male infertility. *Fertility and Sterility* **24**, 802–4.

Shortcliffe, L. M. D., Wehner, N. & Stamey, T. A. (1981) Use of a solid phase radio-immunoassay and formalin-fixed whole bacterial antigen in the detection of antigen-specific immunoglobulin in prostatic fluid. *Journal of Clinical Investigation* **67**, 790–9.

Swenson, C. E., Toth, A. & O'Leary, W. M. (1979) Urea plasma urealyticum and human infertility: The effect of antibiotic therapy on semen quality. *Fertility and Sterility* **31**, 660–5.

Taylor-Robinson, D., Csonka, E. W. & Prentice, M. J. (1977) Human intra-urethral innoculation of urea plasmas. *Quarterly Journal of Medicine* **46**, 309–26.

Teague, N. S., Boyarsky, S. & Glenn, J. F. (1971) Interference of human spermatozoa motility by *Escherichia coli. Fertility and Sterility* **22**, 281–5.

Tuttle, J. P., Holbrook, T. W. & Derrick, F. C. (1977) Intereference of human spermatozoal motility by trichomonas vaginalis. *Journal of Urology* **118**, 1024–5.

13

Diagnosis of Retrograde Ejaculation

Retrograde ejaculation is a fairly common disorder that will cause infertility (Girgis *et al.*, 1968). In this condition, the semen instead of travelling down the penile urethra, passes backwards into the bladder. Patients with this condition will present with absent or very reduced ejaculate (Crich & Jequier, 1978). All patients with infertility and a persistently reduced ejaculatory volume should be suspected of having retrograde ejaculation and investigated accordingly.

Retrograde ejaculation has many causes. Any operation which interferes with the closing mechanism of the bladder neck or the passage of semen down the penile urethra may cause this problem. Neurological disorders can also produce retrograde ejaculation and thus this condition may be seen in spinal injury, diabetes and multiple sclerosis. Retrograde ejaculation may also be the result of the action of drugs on the bladder neck. In patients with this problem it is important to make the diagnosis definitively and to exclude other causes of disordered ejaculation. The diagnosis depends on finding spermatozoa in large numbers in a postcoital urine sample.

Examining a postcoital urine specimen

The patient is asked to have intercourse and then to empty his bladder into a specimen jar. This container needs to be large enough to hold 300–400 ml. The urine may then be brought to the laboratory the following morning.

On arrival at the laboratory, care must be taken to ensure that the urine specimen is well mixed. Urine will kill sperm almost instantaneously. The sperm in this urine specimen will therefore be dead and will sink rapidly to the bottom of the container. In order to identify the sperm and to perform an accurate count, mixing must be very thorough.

After mixing, the volume of the urine is measured and two 10 ml aliquots of urine are removed. The rest of the urine can then be discarded. These 10 ml aliquots are centrifuged, the supernatant removed and the pellets resuspended in 1 ml of phosphate buffer or saline. An estimation of the sperm concentration is then performed in duplicate on each of the sperm suspensions obtained from the two aliquots of urine. Thus from this estimation, the number of sperm present in each of the 10 ml aliquots of urine will be known and the total number of sperm in the urine sample (which will represent the whole ejaculate) may be calculated:

Number of sperm in 10 ml of urine = n

$$\text{Sperm count/ml of urine} = \frac{n}{10}$$

$$\therefore \text{sperm content of ejaculate} = \frac{n}{10} \times \text{volume of urine}$$

The sperm content of the ejaculate is reported as the mean value obtained from two aliquots of urine.

There are, of course, small numbers of sperm left in the urethra after normal antegrade ejaculation. The sperm usually only number a few thousand but will be found in any postcoital urine. The presence of more than 5 million sperm in a postcoital urine makes the presence of retrograde ejaculation very likely.

It is also possible for a patient to have partial retrograde ejaculation (Jequier, unpublished). In these patients, the total sperm count may be obtained by adding the total number of sperm in the urine to those in the reduced volume of antegrade ejaculate.

A diagnostic problem may arise when retrograde ejaculation occurs in a patient who is also azoospermic. In these cases, one must resort to measuring one or more of the seminal markers in a postcoital specimen of urine. Stable compounds which are easy to measure include acid phosphatase and fructose.

Retrograde ejaculation is an easy diagnosis to make and examination of a postcoital urine should form a routine part of a semen analysis service.

References

Crich, J. P. & Jequier, A. M. (1978) Infertility in men with retrograde ejaculation: The action of urine on sperm motility and a simple method for achieving antegrade ejaculation. *Fertility and Sterility* **30**, 572–6.

Girgis, S. M., Etriby, A., El-Hefnawy, H. & Kahil, S. (1968) Aspermia: A survey of 49 cases. *Fertility and Sterility* **19**, 580–8.

14

Tests for Anti-Sperm Antibodies

It has been known since the beginning of this century that sperm can induce an immune response not only between species but also within one species and within an individual. However the possible role of autoimmunity to sperm as a cause of infertility was first described in 1954 when both Rumke and Wilson individually demonstrated the presence of sperm agglutinating and sperm immobilizing antibodies in the sera of a small number of men with infertility. Indeed it was also shown that these patients had spontaneously agglutinating spermatozoa in their semen. There was then found to be a correlation between the presence of autoagglutination of sperm and the absence of penetration of cervical mucus by those sperm. That sperm autoimmunity as a cause of infertility in the human is now well established (Beer & Neaves, 1978) although the exact way by which these antibodies induce infertility is less clear. Sperm antibodies may cause agglutination of sperm, a reduction in motility and inhibit the ability of sperm to penetrate cervical mucus. They may also impede binding of the sperm to the zona pellucida of the oocyte and interfere with the subsequent penetration of the oocyte. It must be remembered that anti-sperm antibodies may also be present in the cervical mucus itself and in this way inhibit the entry of the sperm into the female genital tract. Indeed anti-sperm antibodies may be detected in the female consort from an infertile partnership. Thus immunity to sperm is an important cause of infertility and is a subject which is vital to the proper evaluation of an infertile couple. The detection of anti-sperm antibodies forms an important part of a semen analysis and will be discussed in some detail. There are many ways to detect these antibodies and the most important of these methods are described in this Chapter.

Antigens and their antibodies

The source of antigen for the autoimmune response are the surface antigens of the sperm. These antigens appear to be glycoproteins. However, much cross reactivity appears to occur in relation to the anti-body—antigen reaction. Thus the sites of these antigens cannot neces-sarily be inferred from simple binding studies. Likewise, some anti-sperm antibodies may also cross-react with other human tissues and even bacteria.

The anti-sperm antibodies that are found in blood (humoral anti-bodies) belong to the IgG class but less commonly are also of the IgM and IgA classes. These circulating antibodies reach the semen as a transudate into the secretions of the prostate. Some IgA may also reach the semen in the secretions of the bulbo-urethral glands.

Immunoglobulins of the IgG class are the most common source of anti-sperm antibodies and tend to cause tail-to-tail agglutination of sperm in semen. Much less frequently, immunoglobulins of the IgM class act also as anti-sperm antibodies and these cause head-to-head agglutination of sperm. It is also now known that IgA may be actively secreted into the semen and act as a major sperm agglutinin. However, the level at which these antibodies enter the male reproductive tract is not clear, but sperm agglutinins have been demonstrated even in the epididymal fluid.

The factors that induce the presence of anti-sperm antibodies in serum are varied but it would certainly seem that obstruction of the duct system, either spontaneously or by vasectomy, would appear to in-duce anti-sperm antibody formation (Phadke & Padukone, 1964). Deposits of immune complex have also been found on the walls of the seminiferous tubule and even occasionally on the germ cells them-selves. One must therefore assume that anti-sperm antibodies may induce infertility by causing sperm agglutination; impeding the ability of sperm to pass through cervical mucus; and possibly by interfering with spermatogenesis.

It is now of value to consider some of the ways in which the presence of anti-sperm may be detected either in serum or in the semen itself. There are many tests for anti-sperm antibodies and not all the methods available will be described here. Those tests that are in common use are included in some detail.

Presence of spontaneous sperm agglutination

In some, but not all, patients with anti-sperm antibodies in the semen, agglutination of sperm may occur. This takes place within 10–15 minutes of ejaculation, that is, when the anti-sperm antibodies in the prostatic secretion come into contact with the sperm themselves. The antibodies are polyvalent and join the sperm together causing agglutination (Fig. 14.1). This contact between the spermatozoa can be tail-to-tail, less frequently head-to-head or occasionally a mixture of both. The amount of the sperm that are agglutinated must be made clear for the semen analysis together with the type of agglutination present.

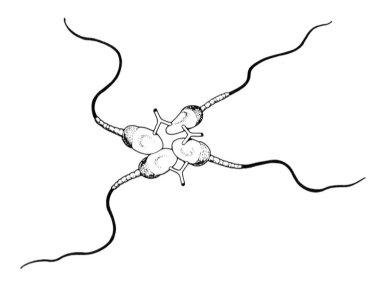

Fig. 14.1. The possible method by which anti-sperm antibodies may cause sperm agglutination.

It is very difficult to assess the numbers of sperm involved in any agglutinated semen (Fig. 14.2). It must also be remembered that it is normal for occasional sperm to stick to debris in semen. It is generally best to decide what percentage of the total spermatozoa are involved in agglutination and report this figure. As such an estimate can only be very approximate, it has been suggested that agglutination may be reported in the following way:

+   less than $\frac{1}{3}$ of total spermatozoa involved in agglutination

+ + $\frac{1}{3}$–$\frac{2}{3}$ of total spermatozoa involved in agglutination

+ + + $\frac{2}{3}$ or more of total spermatozoa involved in agglutination

As it is important to report the type of agglutination as well as the number of sperm involved, a report might read 'Agglutination + +,

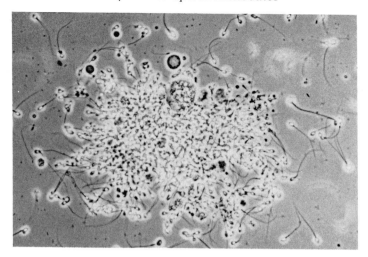

Fig. 14.2. An example of the spontaneous agglutination that may occur in the semen of infertile men.

tail-to-tail'. The small numbers of sperm that are frequently adherent to particulate matter and cellular debris should be ignored and not included on the report.

Methods of demonstrating sperm antibodies

Agglutination tests

As many of the anti-sperm antibodies arrive in the semen only from the circulation, it is clear that methods could be devised to detect their presence in the serum of infertile men. A number of different methods have been described in which the presence of these antibodies is manifested by the ability of the serum to cause agglutination of normal spermatozoa. These tests are simple to perform and are of value clinically but do have the disadvantage that they require a supply of normal fertile human semen.

Gel agglutination test (GAT)

The gel agglutination test was first described by Kibrick *et al.* in 1952 for testing rabbit serum but was later popularized by Shulman (1978) for use in human infertility. The test detects the presence of circulating anti-sperm antibodies of the IgG or IgM classes that can be present in an infertile patient. It can be used to test either male or female sera. If anti-sperm antibodies (which are usually directed against the surface antigens of the sperm) are present in the patient's serum, they will cause normal sperm to agglutinate and clump together as floccules. The serum used in the test must be heat inactivated to re-move complement as the complement reaction will interfere with the sperm flocculation.

The GAT response is simple and cheap to perform but does necessi-tate the use of fairly large volumes of normal semen.

1. *Preparation of the patient's serum*

• The patient's serum is inactivated (freed of complement) by heating at 56°C for 30 minutes.
• The serum is then diluted with Baker's buffer (see Chapter 10). Dilutions of the serum of 1 in 4 and 1 in 20 are often used. As 0.2 ml of the diluted serum will be needed for the test, it is best to make up these dilutions as

> 100 μl of serum in 300 μl of Baker's buffer giving a 1 in 4 dilution, and,
> 50 μl of serum in 950 μl of Baker's buffer producing a 1 in 20 dilution

2. *Preparation of the semen*

• A fresh sample of normal semen is required containing a concentra-tion of sperm of at least 70×10^6/ml and showing good motility of the sperm. An estimate of the sperm concentration in the sample is made and the semen is then diluted with Baker's buffer to produce an approximate sperm concentration of 40×10^6/ml. The sperm suspen-sion is now warmed in a water bath to 37°C.
• A solution of 10% gelatin (Difco Laboratories) is made in Baker's buffer and the solution is also warmed to 37°C.
• An equal volume of the gelatin solution is now added to the sperm suspension and the two mixed carefully by gentle agitation. The gelatin present in the solution enhances the sensitivity of the test.

3. *Incubation of the sperm with the patient's serum*

• The incubation takes place in small glass tubes which should be approximately 3 cm in length and 3 mm in diameter. These tubes can be purchased but can also be made more cheaply in the laboratory by cutting up glass tubing of appropriate diameter and sealing one end.

• A 200 μl aliquot of each of the diluted sera is dispensed into the small glass tubes and then an equal volume (200 μl) of the sperm suspension is added to each tube. The contents are gently mixed.

• The mixture is incubated in a water bath at 37°C for 1 and 2 hours.

• At the end of both the first and second hours, each tube is examined for the presence of sperm flocculation. The tubes are best viewed with lighting from one side against a black card or very dark background. In a positive test, the sperm clump together and form floccules in the lower part of the mixture while the upper part of the solution is cleared (Fig. 14.3).

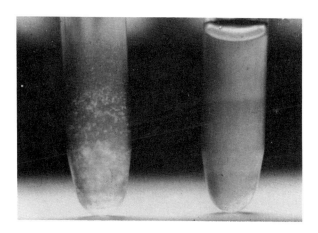

Fig. 14.3. Positive and negative responses in a gel agglutination test.

• It cannot be stressed too strongly, that sera producing known positive and negative responses *must* be included in this assay. It is not difficult to produce either a false negative or a false positive response in this test.

4. Reporting the test

The presence of flocculation in this test is only clinically significant if it is present using serum at dilutions of 1 in 32 or more. Dilutions of 1 in 4 and 1 in 20 are useful for screening as they give one some idea of the 'strength' of the positive reaction. If the test is positive at a dilution of 1 in 20, the serum must be retested at increased dilutions such as 1 in 32, 1 in 64 and 1 in 128 or until a negative test is achieved.

If the test is negative using serum at a dilution of 1 in 32 or less, then the GAT response must be reported to be negative. A positive response at a dilution of 1 in 32 or at a higher dilution is described as positive, and reported to be positive at the greatest dilution at which the positive response was detected.

In this test, massive flocculation of the spermatozoa occurs and it is not possible to determine the type of agglutination (head-to-head or tail-to-tail) that is occurring (Fig. 14.4). However, the advantage of the GAT reaction is that it is simple and easy to perform. Its disadvantage is that it needs relatively large amounts of normal semen. Only around 8–10 samples of serum can be tested in dilutions per sample of normal semen. Thus it may be difficult to obtain such large amounts of normal semen for a laboratory that does not have ready access to a donor insemination programme.

Capillary tube agglutination test

This method, first described by Shulman and Hekman in 1971, uses much finer tubes than does the gel agglutination test but is based on

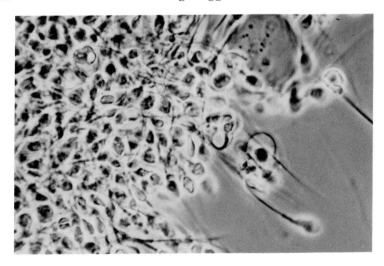

Fig. 14.4. The microscopic appearance of flocculation in a positive gel agglutination test response. It is not possible to determine the type of sperm agglutination that is present.

very similar principles. Moreover, sperm of poor motility may be used in this test. The 10% gelatin solution is also omitted from the mixture and incubation takes place at room temperature. Its great advantage is that much smaller amounts of semen are needed for each test which allows many more sera to be assayed. This method is not frequently employed.

Tray-agglutination test (TAT)

First described by Friberg in 1974, this test is performed in disposable plastic microchambers which are frequently used for tissue culture. This method has the great advantage that only 1 μl of normal semen is needed in each aliquot of serum thus allowing very large numbers of sera to be tested in one batch. However, it is based on the same principles as the gel agglutination test and detects the same class of circulating anti-sperm antibody, though it appears to be a much more sensitive test.

1. *Preparation of the patient's serum*

• The serum to be tested must again be heat inactivated to remove complement by heating to 56°C for 30 minutes.
• The serum to be tested is diluted, this time in 0.01 M phosphate buffered saline at pH 7.4 to produce dilutions of 1 in 4, 1 in 8, 1 in 16 and 1 in 32. These dilutions are maintained at room temperature.

2. *Preparation of the normal semen*

Normal semen containing a fairly high concentration of sperm (at least 70×10^6/ml) is diluted using the 0.01 M phosphate buffered saline at pH 7.4 to produce a sperm concentration of around 40×10^6/ml. This buffer will partially or totally immobilize the sperm.

3. *Incubation of the semen and the diluted sera*

• A 5 μl aliquot of each of the diluted sera is added to the microchambers.
• To this is added a 1 μl aliquot of the sperm suspension. For this addition a Hamilton syringe will be required.
• The mixture is incubated at room temperature for 4 hours.

• At the end of the 4 hour incubation, the contents of the wells of the trays are examined using an inverted microscope at magnification between ×60 and ×600. The degree of agglutination is best seen at low magnification while the type of agglutination is best determined at high magnification.

4. Reporting the test

As with the gel agglutination test, a positive response is clinically significant when present in sera at dilutions of 1 in 32 or more. The lower dilutions are helpful in determining the 'strength' of the positivity of any test and as so little semen is required, large numbers of dilutions can be tested. Using the inverted microscope, the type of agglutination of the sperm can be described.

In order to standardize all reporting of "micro' agglutination tests where both the number of agglutinated sperm can be counted and also the type of agglutination can be assessed, Rose *et al.* (1976) has suggested a method by which the results of these tests should be described. These authors suggest that the degree of agglutination be reported as one of four grades:

1st degree: isolated agglutinate containing <10 sperm with many free sperm
2nd degree: moderate numbers of agglutinate containing 10–15 sperm, some free sperm present
3rd degree: large and plentiful agglutinates each containing >50 sperm, few free sperm
4th degree: gross sperm agglutination, virtually no free sperm.

The agglutination must also be reported qualitatively and four types of sperm agglutination may be seen. These are:

Head-to-head (often due to IgM)
Tail-to-tail (often due to IgG)
Tailtip-Tailtip
Tangle (heads and tails adherent where it is difficult to define a specific type)

This method for reporting sperm agglutination in an agglutination test is depicted diagrammatically in Fig. 14.5. Although theoretically such a method of description could be used in relation to spontaneous sperm agglutination, the clumping of sperm in this situation is usually too excessive to be amenable to any accurate descriptive analysis.

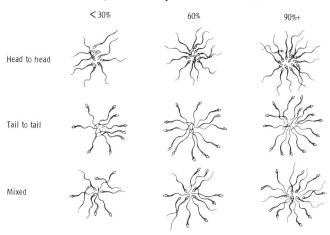

Fig. 14.5. A diagrammatic representation of the type and extent of sperm agglutination that may be seen in a micro-agglutination test.

Tube-slide agglutination test (TSAT)

Another way of detecting the presence of anti-sperm antibodies in a patient's serum is the tube-slide agglutination test. This test is best used for testing female sera. It is simply an extension of the slide test first described by Rumpke and Hellinga in 1959. The tube-slide agglutination test was first reported by Franklin and Dukes in 1964 and has often been known as the Franklin–Dukes Test. More recently, the method has been modified and one of the more commonly used modifications will be described here.

The tube-slide agglutination test is rather more cumbersome and time-consuming than the other agglutination tests described so far but it only requires small volumes of semen and it is also possible that it is detecting antibodies present in the serum that may not produce a positive response in either the gel or the tray agglutination tests.

1. *Preparation of the patient's serum*

• The serum must first be inactivated and rid of complement by heating to 56°C for 30 minutes.
• The serum is now diluted 1 in 4 with Baker's buffer.

2. *Preparation of the semen*

A fresh sample of semen containing sperm of good motility is diluted to produce a sperm concentration of around 50×10^{6}/ml.

3. *Incubation of the serum and semen*

• Into a small test tube is placed 0.5 ml of the diluted serum.
• To this is added a 0.05 µl aliquot of the diluted semen sample. The diluted serum and the sperm suspension are mixed using gentle agitation. It is probably best to perform each test in duplicate as in this method only one dilution of serum is used.
• The mixture is incubated at 37°C and examined at 1 and 2 hours.
• After 1 and 2 hours of incubation a drop is removed from each tube and examined microscopically.

4. *Reporting the test*

At microscopy, the number of motile cells in each of 12 high power fields are counted. The number of motile clumped sperm are also counted. The total number of motile clumped sperm is divided by the total number of motile cells and multiplied by 100. Thus the percentage of motile clumped sperm are estimated. The test is deemed to be positive if more than 10% of the motile sperm are clumped.

It is also important to include in the report the type of sperm agglutination that is occurring in this test.

Sperm immobilizing antibody test (SIT)

In the sera of some infertile patients, there are antibodies which cause the immobilization (loss of motility) of spermatozoa. These antibodies interact with the surface of the sperm and are, unlike the agglutination tests, complement dependant. These antibodies are only of the IgM and IgG classes as IgA does not activate complement.

This test was first introduced by both Fjallbrant in 1968 and also by Isojima *et al.* in the same year. Both methods are very similar, but only the more commonly used Isojima method will be described here.

Isojima sperm immobilizing test

For this test, control sera, guinea pig serum, normal human serum, rabbit anti-human sperm serum and normal semen containing sperm showing good motility are used.

1. *Preparation of sera*

• Serum is needed from normal humans (which contains no immobilizing activity) to act as a control. This serum is inactivated and complement removed by heating to 56°C for 30 minutes.
• The test sera from the infertile patients is also inactivated by heating to 56°C for 30 minutes.
• Rabbit anti-human sperm serum (RAS) which is available commercially, is appropriately diluted in saline so that it will immobilize at least 90–95% of sperm in the presence of complement. This dilution may be known if the serum is obtained commercially but if the serum is prepared in an on-site laboratory and animal house, the necessary dilution of the serum must first be ascertained before use in the sperm immobilizing test. A small amount of guinea pig serum must also be rendered complement free by heating, as this will be used to detect any non-complement dependent immobilizing activity that could be present in the guinea pig serum.

2. *Preparation of the semen*

Normal semen containing sperm at a concentration of at least 60×10^6/ml with a motility of more than 70% and also demonstrating good forward progression, is diluted in normal saline to produce a concentration of sperm of around 60×10^6/ml. An *accurate* estimate of the motility is now made.

3. *Preparation of the complement source*

Complement is present in the guinea pig serum. There are many commercial preparations of complement in guinea pig sera in which the content of complement is known. The guinea pig serum is usually stored at -20°C in small aliquots as repeated freezing and thawing will damage the activity of the complement in serum.

4. *Incubation of sera, complement and semen*

The incubation is carried out in small tubes such as those used in serological laboratories.

• To each tube is added 25 μl of physiological saline, 25 μl of inactivated normal human saline, 25 μl of rabbit anti-sperm antibody serum and 25 μl of the serum under test. It is best to perform each test in duplicate.

• To all but one pair of tubes is added 50 μl of the complement source, that is, the guinea pig serum. Into the remaining pair of tubes is added a 50 μl aliquot of guinea pig serum that has been heat inactivated.

• The samples are now incubated at 32°C for 1 hour, after which the sperm are examined microscopically and the percentage motility reliably estimated.

5. *Reporting the test*

If the motility of the sperm has been reduced to one half or less of the original motility, then the test is reported as 'positive'. Sera which give a positive response may be tested in dilutions which are usually performed in serial two-fold dilutions up to 1 in 128.

This sperm immobilizing test seeks the presence of antibodies that are not demonstrated by the complement-independent agglutination test. This test is particularly helpful in detecting the presence of anti-sperm antibodies in infertile women especially those who show no invasion of sperm into the cervical mucus as such antibodies may be found in the cervico-vaginal secretions of infertile women.

However, the sperm immobilization test is subject to artefact and it is very important that the protocol is carefully adhered to and rigid control systems are incorporated into the assay.

6. *Quantitating the test*

It is also possible to quantitate the response in the sperm immobilization test (Rose *et al.*, 1976). For this a standard curve must be produced using the sperm immobilizing activity of a standard serum. This methodology is useful for research but is not usually employed in a routine laboratory.

The sperm immobilizing test is of value in the evaluation of immune infertility but is probably not necessary as a routine test. It can be applied to special types of immunological problems that may cause infertility.

Test for cytotoxic antibodies

In this test described by Hamerlynk and Rumke (1968) the presence of damage to the sperm by complement is not tested by determining a reduction in motility but by the ability of dyes to stain the spermatozoa whose plasma membranes have been breeched. In this protocol, the inactivated serum, a complement source and normal spermatozoa are incubated with eosin and trypan blue. The percentage of stained cells is then counted.

The procedure frequently used is a modification (Rose *et al.*, 1976) of the original method described by Hamerlynk and Rumpke (1968). It is this modification that will be described.

For the sperm cytotoxicity test, normal semen, guinea pig serum (as a source of complement), formalin and trypan blue is needed.

1. *Preparation of the semen*

A fresh sample of semen with a known sperm concentration of at least 60×10^6/ml is diluted 1 in 10 with phosphate buffered saline (PBS) at pH 7.4 and centrifuged at 50 G for 30 minutes. The supernatant is aspirated and the sediment resuspended in PBS to produce a sperm concentration of 100×10^6/ml. The sperm are washed in this way in order to remove any anti-complement factors that can be present in seminal plasma.

2. *Preparation of the sera*

The patient's serum for testing must first be inactivated by heating to 56°C for 30 minutes. Known positive and negative sera *must* be included as controls.

The guinea pig serum which has been stored in frozen aliquots is thawed for use in this test. This is then diluted to 1 in 10 with PBS. The exact dilution of the guinea pig serum used will depend on its content of complement.

3. *Preparation of formalin and the trypan blue*

A 30% solution of formalin is needed for this assay. A 1% solution of trypan blue is made up in PBS.

4. *Incubation of the semen and sera*

• Using small tubes (e.g., LP3 tubes) 0.1 ml of the inactivated sera under test is added to the tube followed by 0.05 ml of the sperm suspension (which contains 50×10^6 sperm/ml). They are incubated at 37°C for 30 minutes.
• To the incubate is added 0.3 ml of the diluted guinea pig sera and the mixture is now incubated at the lower temperature of 30°C for a further 30 minutes.
• To this mixture is added 50 μl of the 1% solution of trypan blue. The temperature of the water bath is raised again to 37°C and the mixture incubated for another 30 minutes.
• A 300 μl aliquot of 30% formalin is added to the mixture as this will break up any sperm aggregates.
• The sperm are now examined microscopically and a direct count is made of the stained and unstained cells which represent undamaged and damaged cells.

5. *Reporting the test*

The total cells counted must contain at least 100 unstained cells. Thus the total number of cells = 100 + number of stained cells. The result of the cytotoxicity test is usually reported as the 'spermocytotoxicity index' (STI) = 100 − number of stained cells. For this reason, the complement concentration in the assay must allow there to be more unstained than stained cells.

Other techniques used to demonstrate cytotoxicity

It is also possible to use a microtechnique (Rose *et al.*, 1976) which combines both an immobilization and a cytotoxicity test in one assay. This test has the advantage that only a small amount of semen is needed and thus large numbers of sera can be tested. It also has the advantage that the responses can be quantitated. It is, however, in routine use in only a few laboratories.

Recently a more sophisticated approach to the cytotoxic test has been described. Suominen *et al.* (1980) determined the reduction in ATP release from the damaged cells in relation to a control as a means of defining cytotoxicity. In 1981, Mathur *et al.* described a double staining technique so that the dead and alive sperm could easily be differentiated in the cytotoxicity test. The usefulness of these new tests remains to be evaluated.

Mixed antiglobulin reaction (MAR test)

This method was originally described by Coombs in 1973 but perfected by Jager *et al.* in 1978 and put into routine use by Hendry and Stedronska in 1980. It detects the presence of antibody on the surface of the sperm themselves. It has the great advantage that it detects both IgG and IgA on sperm and is simple to perform. It does not require samples of normal fertile semen. It has the disadvantage, as it detects the antibody on the patient's sperm, of being applicable only indirectly to azoospermic men.

In this test, red blood cells are coated with IgA or sensitized with IgG. These cells are then mixed with a monospecific anti IgA or an anti IgG. These treated red cells are then incubated with the sperm under test. If the sperm carry anti-sperm antibodies of the appropriate class, then they will adhere to the red blood cells (Fig. 14.6).

1. *Preparation of the red blood cells*

• Group O rhesus positive blood is needed and this can either be purchased or more easily obtained from a haematological laboratory. Approximately 5 ml of blood is sufficient to test 30 semen samples.
• To this blood is added an equal volume of Alsever's solution (Table 14.1) and the two solutions mixed and then centrifuged. The supernatant is then decanted and discarded. The red cells are washed with Alsever's solution twice more in the same way.
• After the third centrifugation and removal of the supernatant, a sufficient volume of Alsever's solution is added to equal the volume of the red blood cell pellet at the bottom of the tube. This will produce a 50% suspension of red blood cells in Alsever's solution.

2. *Preparation of the human serum*

• Human venous blood is placed in a glass tube and allowed to clot and

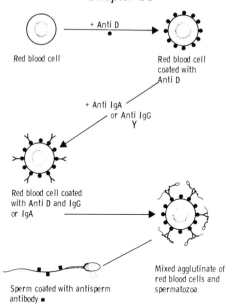

Red blood cell

Red blood cell
coated with
Anti D

+ Anti D

+ Anti IgA
or Anti IgG

Red blood cell coated
with Anti D and IgG
or IgA

Mixed agglutinate of
red blood cells and
spermatozoa

Sperm coated with antisperm
antibody ■

Fig. 14.6. A diagrammatic representation of the MAR test.

Table 14.1. The formulation of Alsever's
solution for use in the MAR test

Dextrose	20.5 g
Sodium Citrate	8.0 g
Citric Acid	0.552 g
Sodium Chloride	4.2 g
Distilled water to make up to 1 litre	

to stand at room temperature for 2 hours. The tube is then centrifuged
and the supernatant removed. The remaining clot is discarded.
• The serum is diluted to 1 in 5 in distilled water.
• A preparation of anti-D (usually 'fortified anti-D' available from the
National Blood Transfusion Service) is added to the diluted serum to
produce itself a dilution of 1 in 20 in the diluted serum.
• Two parts of the diluted serum (containing the anti-D) is added to
1 part of the red blood cell suspension and the mixture is incubated at

37°C for 30 minutes. The cells thus become coated with anti-D. This mixture can be prepared in bulk as it can be stored at 4°C for up to 1 month. Thus for everyday use, the MAR test only involves the protocol outlined below.

3. *Incubation of the coated red cells and the spermatozoa*

• 1 drop of the semen under test is placed on a microscope slide and to it is added 1 drop of the sensitized cells and mixed.
• 1 drop of an undiluted anti-human globulin raised against either IgG or IgA is now added to the mixture.
• The mixture *must* be examined within 10 minutes (5 minutes is best) and the number of motile sperm which have adhered to the red cells are assessed. The MAR test is depicted diagrammatically in Fig. 14.6.

4. *Reporting the test*

The test is reported as positive or negative, that is, the presence or absence of motile sperm adherent to the red cells which thus form mixed agglutinates to sperm and red blood cells is reported. The results are often reported numerically but it is important to give an estimate of the percentage of the motile sperm that are adherent to the red blood cells as is demonstrated below:

'0' = Negative   = no motile mixed agglutinates, all sperm swimming freely, occasional non-motile mixed agglutinates
'1' = Positive   = 10–90% of the motile sperm form mixed agglutinates
'2' = Strongly positive = 90–100% of the motile sperm are attached to the red blood cells, very few freely motile sperm

The test is probably clinically relevant when more than 50% of the motile sperm are adherent to the red blood cells. The MAR test has the great advantage that as the sensitized red cells can be prepared for up to a month in advance and the incubation of the red cells with the spermatozoa only lasts 5 minutes, this test can be performed with ease on all semen samples which contain motile sperm that are sent to the laboratory. As it detects the presence of the clinically important anti-sperm antibodies of the IgG and IgA classes on the surface of the sperm (depending on the anti-globulin used) it is of great value in the assessment of the potential fertility of a specimen of semen.

The MAR test can also be performed indirectly by incubating normal sperm with the seminal fluid from azoospermic men. If anti-sperm antibodies are present in the azoospermic semen, the normal sperm will become coated with them and so produce a positive result in a MAR test. The authors believe that the MAR test should probably be used routinely on all semen brought to the laboratory for evaluation.

Indirect and direct sperm immunofluorescence

Using the technique of immunofluorescence, it is possible to demonstrate the presence of anti-sperm antibodies in the sera of patients by applying the serum to normal spermatozoa (indirect method) and then staining these sperm with a fluorescein conjugated anti-globulin preparation (Hjort & Hansen, 1971). It is also possible to demonstrate the presence of anti-sperm antibodies that are already on the surface of the sperm by simple staining with the conjugate (direct technique).

1. *Preparation of the sperm*

• Sperm either from a normal donor (indirect method) or from the patient under test (direct method) are washed twice in normal saline and separated each time by centrifugation at 680 G for 5 minutes. About 0.2 ml of semen is washed with 10 ml of saline provided that the semen has a reasonable sperm concentration.
• After the second wash the sperm are resuspended in saline, the volume being adjusted to produce a sperm concentration of around 10×10^6/ml.
• Single drops of this suspension are spread onto clean glass sides and air-dried with a fan for 30 minutes.
• The sperm are now fixed in absolute alcohol (analytical grade) for 30 minutes and then transferred in PBS at pH 7.2.

Indirect method only
• After wiping off the excess moisture with a tissue, a drop of serum is placed on top of the smear and the slide incubated in a micro chamber for 1 hour at around 20°C.
• The serum is then rinsed of with the PBS and washed for 20 minutes in two changes of buffer.

Direct and indirect methods — staining the slide
• To the dry smear is now added a fluorescein conjugated antiserum. These sera are easily available commercially and can be directed against one or more of the immunoglobulin classes. The antiserum is incubated on the slide for 30 minutes also at room temperature.
• After repeated washing in the PBS, the slide is mounted in a solution of PBS containing 10% glycerol.
• The presence of fluorescence is then sought using a fluorescent microscope.

This technique is beset by non-specific staining. If non-specificity can be excluded, areas of immunofluorescence may be seen to involve the whole or only part of the spermatozoa. The immunoglobulin classes IgM and IgG are most commonly found to coat sperm using this method but the IgA class is known to produce fluorescence particularly in the region of the equatorial segment of the sperm.

Antibodies that are present but are directed against internal antigens of sperm may also be detected by indirect immunofluorescence using a technique described using rat sperm by Kolk *et al.* in 1974. In this method, the sperm are first treated with dithiothretal in Tris-HCl which causes the sperm heads to swell and exposes the nuclear proteins. How relevant this technique is to human infertility is still not certain.

Sperm-cervical mucus contact test (SCMC)

It is well known that infertility can be induced by the presence of anti-sperm antibodies in the secretions of the genital tract of the female partner and the cervical mucus is an important site for these sperm specific immunoglobulins. These antibodies are usually of the IgA class but immunoglobulins of the IgG class may also be responsible for this type of infertility. These anti-sperm antibodies may manifest themselves in cervical mucus by interfering with the movement of sperm through that mucus (Kremer & Jager, 1976). It is believed that the anti-sperm antibody that may be present in the cervical mucus will cause the sperm to become attached to the strands of the mucoprotein known as micelles, within the ovulatory mucus, and thus impede the forward movement of the sperm. The sperm cannot progress forward but they remain motile and produce what is known as the 'shaking phenomenon'. This abnormal movement has been shown by Kremer and Jager (1980) to be dependent on the presence of a sperm specific immunoglobulin usually of the IgA class within the cervical mucus.

1. *Preparation of the semen*

A semen sample is placed in an upright test tube and allowed to stand at room temperature for 30 minutes, thus letting all the agglutinated and dead sperm sink to the bottom.

2. *Preparation of the cervical mucus*

Preovulatory cervical mucus is aspirated into a quill and a drop of this mucus is placed on a clean glass slide.

3. *Sperm-cervical mucus contact*

• A 100 µl aliquot of the semen is removed from just below the surface of the semen sample and is placed on the slide in contact with the cervical mucus. The mucus and the semen are then mixed on the slide and the mixture is lightly covered with a glass coverslip. A second drop of the semen is placed on the same slide, out of contact with the mucus and also covered with a coverslip.
• The slide is then placed in a Petri dish and incubated at room temperature for 30 minutes.
• Both areas of the slide are then examined microscopically. The area containing semen alone can be used to demonstrate that the 'shaking phenomenon' does not occur spontaneously. If it does occur in the sperm in contact with the cervical mucus, then it can only be caused by the cervical mucus.

This is a quick and very useful test in the evaluation of the fertility potential of semen.

Other new techniques

A technique by which radioimmunoassay has been employed to detect the presence of anti-sperm antibodies bound to the cell surface has now been described by Han and Tung (1979). Other assays described include the measurement of Fc receptors for IgG on sperm and also the use of a solid phase micro-radioimmunoassay used to measure anti-sperm antibodies quantitatively (Mathur *et al.*, 1981).

More recently the 'ELISA' technique has also been applied to the measurement of anti-sperm antibodies (Ing *et al.*, 1985). Another method using 'immunobeads' where polyacrylamide beads coated with antiglobulin may be shown to adhere to sperm that are coated with specific anti-sperm antibody has recently been described (Clarke *et al.*, 1985).

Summary

The choice of a method for the detection of sperm antibodies will depend on the facilities available within each individual laboratory. It is, however, important to use a test that detects all the three main classes of immunoglobulin (Table 14.2). It is likely however that the MAR test and a micro-agglutination method or tray agglutination test will be the methods of choice of most laboratories. The agglutination tests screen for all classes of agglutinating antibodies. In the tray test, for example, semen is used in very small amounts and can therefore be used to test large numbers of sera in many dilutions. The MAR test is simple, does not require normal semen and can be used to test all semen that contain spermatozoa. However, using normal sperm, it can also be used to test azoospermic semen for the presence of antibodies. Some tests for the presence of anti-sperm antibodies should form part of the service provided by a laboratory to a fertility clinic. The tests used to detect the presence or absence of anti-sperm antibodies should be almost as an important part of the male fertility work up as is the semen analysis.

Table 14.2. The anti-sperm antibody tests and the classes of immunoglobulin that they detect

Test	Immuoglobulin Class
Agglutination tests	
GAT	
TAT	IgG, IgM, IgA
TSAT	
Sperm immobilization tests	IgG, IgM
Spermo cytotoxicity tests	IgG, IgM
Kremer test	IgA (occasionally IgG)
MAR	IgG, IgA

References

Beer, A. E. & Neaves, W. B. (1978) Antigenic status of semen from the viewpoints of the female and male. *Fertility and Sterility* **29**, 3–22.

Clarke, E. N., Stojanoff, A., Cauchie, M. N. & Johnstone, W. I. M. (1985) The Immunological Class of Antispermatozool Antibodies in Serum. *American Journal of Reproductive Immunology and Microbiology* **7**, 143–7.

Coombs, R. R. A., Rümpke, P. & Edwards, R. G. (1973) Immunoglobulin classes reactive with spermatozoa in the serum and seminal plasma of vasectomised and infertile men. In Bratamov, K. (ed.) *Proceedings of the Second International Symposium on Immunology of Reproduction*, pp. 354–9. Bulgarian Academy of Science Press.

Fjallbrant, B. (1968) Inter-relation between high levels of sperm antibodies, reduced penetration of cervical mucus by spermatozoa and sterility in men. *Acta Obstetrica Gynecologica Scandinavica* **47**, 102–8.

Franklin, R. R. & Dukes, C. D. (1964) Antispermatozoal activity and unexplained infertility. *American Journal of Obstetrics and Gynecology* **89**, 6–9.

Friberg, J. (1974) A simple and sensitive micromethod for demonstration of sperm agglutinating activity in serum from infertile men and women. *Acta Obstetrica Gynecologica Scandinavica* (Suppl) **36**, 21–19.

Hamerlynck, J. V. T. H. & Rumke, P. (1968) A test for the detection of cytotoxic antibodies to spermatozoa in man. *Journal of Reproduction and Fertility* **17**, 191–4.

Han, L. P. B. & Tung, K. (1979) A quantitative assay for antibodies to surface antigens of guinea pig testicular cells and spermatozoa. *Biology and Reproduction* **21**, 99–107.

Hendry, W. F. & Stedronska, J. (1980) Mixed erythrocyte-spermatozoa antiglobulin reaction (MAR) test for IgA antisperm antibodies in subfertile males. *Journal of Obstetrics and Gynaecology* **1**, 59–62.

Hjort, T. & Hansen, K. B. (1971) Immunofluorescent studies on human spermatozoa. II. Characterisation of spermatozoal antigens and their occurrence in spermatozoa from the male partners of infertile couples. *Clinical and Experimental Immunology* **8**, 9–23.

Ing, R. M. Y., Wang, S-X., Brenneke, A. M. & Jones, W. R. (1985) An improved Indirect Enzyme-Linked Immunosorbent Assay (ELISA) for the detection of antisperm antibodies. *American Journal of Reproductive Immunology and Microbiology* **8**, 15–19.

Isojima, S., Li, T. S. & Ashitaka, Y. (1968) Immunologic analysis of sperm immobilising factor found in sera of women with unexplained infertility. *American Journal of Obstetrics and Gynecology* **101**, 677–83.

Jager, S., Kremer, J. & Van Slochteren-Draaisma, T. (1978) A simple method of screening for antisperm antibodies in the male. Detection of spermatozoal surface IgG with the direct mixed antiglobulin reaction carried out on untreated fresh human semen. *International Journal of Infertility* **23**, 12–21.

Kibrick, S., Belding, D. L. & Merrill, B. (1952) Methods for the detection of antibodies against mammalian spermatozoa: Gelatin Agglutination Test. *Fertility and Sterility* **3**, 419–38.

Kolk, A. H. J., Samuel, T. & Rumke, P. (1974) Autoantigens of human spermatozoa. I. Solubilisation of a new autoantigen detected on swollen sperm heads. *Clinical and Experimental Immunology* **16**, 63–76.

Kremer, J. & Jager, S. (1976) The Sperm-Cervical Mucus Contact Test: A preliminary report. *Fertility and Sterility* **27**, 335–40.

Kremer, J. & Jager, S. (1980) Characterisation of anti-spermatozoal antibodies responsible for the shaking phenomenon with special regard to immunoglobin class and antigen-reactive sites. *International Journal of Andrology* **3**, 143–52.

Mathur, S., Williamson, H. O., Derrick, F. C., Madyastha, P. R., Melchers, J. T., Hotz, G. L., Baker, E. R., Smith, C. L. & Fudenberg, H. H. (1981) A new microassay for spermatotoxic antibody: Comparison with passive hemagglutination assay for anti-sperm antibodies in couples with unexplained infertility. *Journal of Immunology* **126**, 905–9.

Phadke, A. M. & Padukone, K. (1964) Presence and significance of auto-antibodies against spermatozoa in the blood of men with obstructed vas deferens. *Journal of Reproduction and Fertility* **7**, 162–70.

Rose, N. R., Hjort, J., Rumke, P., Harper, M. J. K. & Vyazov, O. (1976) Techniques for detection of iso- and auto-antibodies to human spermatozoa. *Clinical and Experimental Immunology* **23**, 175–99.

Rumke, P. (1954) The presence of sperm antibodies in the serum of two patients with oligozoospermia. *Vox Sang* (Basel) **4**, 135–40.

Rumke, P. & Hellinga, G. (1959) Autoantibodies against spermatozoa in sterile men. *American Journal of Clinical Pathology* **32**, 357–63.

Shulman, S. (1978) Agglutinating and immobilising antibodies to spermatozoa. In Cohen, J. & Hendry, W. F. (eds), *Spermatozoa, Antibodies and Infertility* pp. 81–99. Blackwell Scientific Publications, Oxford.

Shulman, S. & Hekman, A. (1971) Antibodies to spermatozoa. I. A new macroscopic agglutination technique for their detection, using immotile sperm. *Clinical and Experimental Immunology* **9**, 137–46.

Suominen, J. J. O., Multamaki, S. & Djupsund, B. M. (1980) A new method for measurement of cytotoxic antibodies to human spermatozoa. *Archives of Andrology* **4**, 257–64.

Wilson, L. (1954) Spermagglutinins in human semen and blood. *Proceedings of the Society of Experimental Biology and Medicine* **85**, 652–5.

15

Sperm Function Tests

During the course of a semen analysis, the spermatozoa are examined in many different ways. The number, the motility and the morphology of the sperm are examined and their structure is sometimes demonstrated in the very great detail that is achieved by electron microscopy. However, until now, no attempt has been made to test the ability of spermatozoa to perform the function for which each is designed, namely penetrating cervical mucus, entering the female genital tract, traversing the genital tract and penetrating an oocyte. Many of these functions can indeed be tested within the laboratory. Such procedures are known as sperm function tests and will be described below.

Testing the ability of sperm to penetrate cervical mucus

The ability of spermatozoa to penetrate cervical mucus and also the ability of cervical mucus to be penetrated by sperm may be tested both *in vivo* and also, in much greater detail, *in vitro*.

Normally cervical mucus is only penetrable by sperm around the time of ovulation. As ovulation approaches, the action of the oestrogen that is being produced by the developing follicle increases the amount of mucus, improves its elasticity or so-called 'spinnbarkeit' (Fig. 15.1) and causes the micelles within the mucus to straighten (Odeblad, 1968) and allow the passage of the spermatozoa through the mucus (Fig. 15.2). Thus any method that is used to test the interaction between sperm and mucus, must only involve the use of ovulatory mucus or mucus from a patient who has been treated with oestrogen.

Postcoital test

This test was first described by Sims more than 100 years ago and is now known either as the Sims or the Sims-Huhner test. A patient is

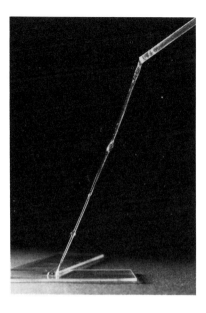

Fig. 15.1. Ovulatory cervical mucus showing the elasticity known as 'Spinnbarkeit'.

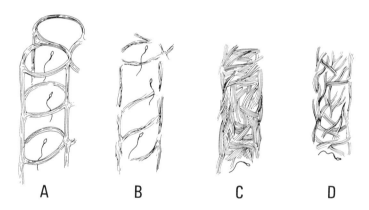

Fig. 15.2. Some of the changes in the arrangement of the micelles within the cervical mucus that takes place during the course of the menstrual cycle.

asked to have intercourse within 48 hours of ovulation, and then come to the clinic 2–6 hours later. At the clinic, the mucus is aspirated and examined microscopically for the presence of motile sperm. The test can be graded according to the number of motile sperm showing forward progression per high power field but is usually reported as the mean number of motile sperm seen in a high power field. This test indeed correlates well with pregnancy rates but pregnancy will occur in many patients with a negative postcoital test and conversely women with positive tests can remain infertile. However the one advantage of the postcoital test is that at least it demonstrates that sexual intercourse is taking place.

The greatest problem with the postcoital test is timing: even in normally ovulating women, the postcoital test may only remain positive for 2–3 days around ovulation. Careful monitoring of ovulation in relation to a postcoital test may give results that correlate in the future more fully with fertility.

In vitro invasion tests

The ability of sperm to penetrate ovulatory cervical mucus can be tested very easily *in vitro*. The cervical mucus is aspirated from the cervical canal at mid cycle close to the time of ovulation. It is best aspirated into a quill or a specially produced plastic capillary aspirator (Rocket of London Ltd). The sperm invasion test can be carried out in a number of different ways.

Slide technique

The mucus is laid out on a clean glass slide. Care must be taken to avoid disruption on the linearity of the micelles within the mucus (Fig. 15.3). A coverslip is now dropped onto the mucus, making sure that no excessive pressure is applied to the mucus. The semen then comes into contact with the mucus only when the mucus is under the coverslip. The technique of applying the coverslip to the mucus *before* there is any contact between it and the semen, prevents sperm coming to lie on top of the mucus which may thus produce a false positive result. The preparation should be examined at 0, 5, 30, 60 and 180 minutes. In normal patients, rapid invasion of the mucus should occur and large numbers of actively motile sperm should be in the mucus within 15 minutes (Fig. 15.4).

Capillary tube technique

This technique was first described by Kremer (1965) and involves the aspiration of mucus into capillary tubes. It is simple to set up this

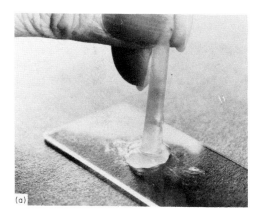

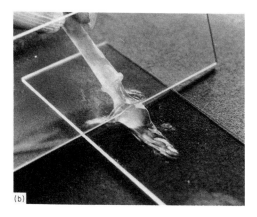

Fig. 15.3. (a) The wrong and (b) the right way to apply cervical mucus to a slide.

apparatus (Fig. 15.5). A glass slide is graduated by scoring millimetre marks along one side using a diamond pen. A sperm reservoir is now made by halving the lower end of a 0.5 cm test tube and glueing one half to the graduated slide. This reservoir is filled with the semen under test. The ovulatory mucus which must show a good 'spinnbarkeit' (elasticity), is aspirated into a wide bore capillary tube. One end of the capillary tube with the mucus protruding slightly (so as to produce good contact with the sperm) is placed in the semen and the tube layed between the supports on the slide. The far end of the capillary tube is sealed with a non-toxic wax. The mounted tube is now laid horizontally in a Petri dish together with some moistened filter

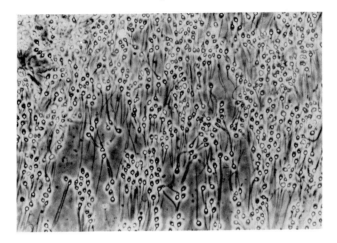

Fig. 15.4. Rapid and spectacular invasion of ovulatory cervical mucus by spermatozoa. Note the presence of each 'phalanx' of spermatozoa as they pass up between the micelles in the mucus. The micelles can only be visualized using electron microscopy. From Jequier, A. M. (1986). In *Scientific Foundations of Obstetrics and Gynaecology*, p. 85, Phillip, E. E., Barnes, J. & Newton, M. (eds). William Heinemann, London.

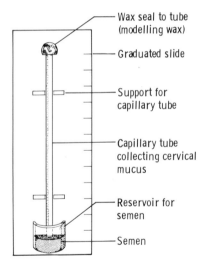

Wax seal to tube
(modelling wax)

Graduated slide

Support for
capillary tube

Capillary tube
collecting cervical
mucus

Reservoir for
semen

Semen

Fig. 15.5. The use of a tube containing cervical mucus into which the penetration by spermatozoa can be tested. This method was described by Kremer (1965).

paper to provide humidity and incubated at 37°C for 1 hour. The capillary tube is now examined microscopically and the distance travelled by the sperm up the tube is ascertained. This distance travelled by the vanguard of sperm is measured in millimetres. If good mucus is used, sperm should be able to travel at least 50 mm in 1 hour.

Crossed invasion or crossed hostility test

In order that cervical mucus may be successfully entered and traversed by spermatozoa, two important factors must be present. Firstly, as has already been discussed, the spermatozoa must be actively motile and be capable of passing up the mucus between the micelles. Secondly, the mucus itself must be ovulatory and must itself contain no other impediments to the entry and the passage of spermatozoa. Thus if during a sperm invasion test, the sperm fail to enter the mucus (or die upon entry) it may be difficult to decide whether it is the sperm or the mucus or both that is at fault. This problem can be sorted out by the use of a crossed invasion test. In this test the husband's sperm and also sperm from a known fertile donor are tested against the infertile wife's mucus. Likewise the husband's sperm and sperm from a donor of known fertility may be tested for invasion against mucus from an ovulatory woman of known fertility or against some bovine mucus or mucus substitute (Fig. 15.6). In this way all the factors that may interfere with sperm penetration of cervical mucus may be elicited.

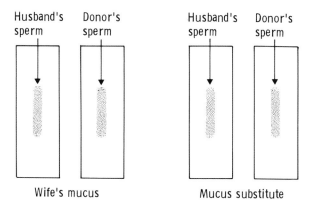

Fig. 15.6. A diagrammatic representation of a 'crossed invasion' test.

1. *Wife's cervical mucus*

The penetration of the wife's mucus in a crossed invasion test does depend on the availability of fertile semen. If semen from a sperm bank is freely available, then this test is easy to perform. If however fertile semen is only occasionally available, the mucus can be stored at $-18°C$ for several weeks until a specimen of fertile semen is available.

The invasion test may be performed using the slide or the capillary method. If the husband's sperm fail to penetrate the wife's mucus but the donor sperm enter the mucus freely, this is likely to be due to a problem in the semen. If neither the husband's nor the donor sperm enter the wife's mucus, this is very probably due to the presence of a barrier in the mucus, but one cannot exclude a concurrent problem of mucus penetration by the husband's sperm. This latter possibility is answered by testing sperm penetration into mucus from another female patient or by testing penetration by the sperm into some form of mucus substitute.

2. *Donor mucus or human cervical mucus substitute*

The husband's semen is now tested with a semen sample of known fertility for its ability to invade mucus of known penetrability. This mucus may be taken from an ovulatory woman at midcycle but the collection of such samples is very time-consuming and also may require special attendance by specific patients. This procedure, using donor mucus is not really very practical except in special circumstances.

One may therefore consider the use of human mucus substitutes for this purpose. The most commonly used human mucus substitute is bovine mucus (Alexander, 1981), obtainable from farms or agricultural institutes. It may be cut up into small strips and each 'aliquot' placed in a small lidded container (Bijou tube) and stored at $-18°C$ until needed. Bovine mucus has all the characteristics of human mucus and thus can be used as a mucus substitute with confidence. Bovine mucus was once available as a commercial preparation and marketed as a thin layer of mucus on a slide. Sadly, this useful, though relatively costly preparation, is no longer available. Another natural substance that may be used as a mucus substitute is egg white. Only very fresh eggs of less than 48 hours old should be utilized, and only that part of the white closest to the yolk used for testing sperm penetration. This mucus substitute may be easily obtainable for some country based laboratories but may be much more of a problem for a semen analysis laboratory situated in the centre of a large city. Experiments are under way to assess the possibility of using synthetic substances as mucus substitutes and the one most tested in this respect is Polyacrylamide gel (PAG). This substance is available in many laboratories and thus may be of use but PAG has the disadvantage that after hydration it may become toxic to sperm and so produce false negative invasion tests. Recently, however, a hyaluronic acid preparation known as *Healon* (Pharmacia Pharmaceuticals) also has some promise as a mucus substitute.

Thus the use of the crossed invasion test is advantageous diagnostically but the necessary 'reagents' may be difficult to obtain for a large number of laboratories.

The 'shaking phenomenon'

This phenomenon was first reported by Kremer and Jager (1976) and may be a manifestation of the presence of anti-sperm antibodies either in the seminal plasma or in the cervical mucus itself. It has already been described in Chapter 13. The sperm enter the mucus but thereafter show no forward progression. The sperm still stay in one place and show motility but no forward movement of the head occurs. It appears that the immunoglobulins of the IgA class may be of importance here. The 'shaking phenomenon' may well be seen during an invasion test and must be recognized.

Laparoscopic sperm retrieval

This is not a very frequently used sperm function test and is one that is performed by the clinician. It assesses the ability of the spermatozoa to enter and to traverse the female genital tract (Templeton & Mortimer, 1982). Infertile women at midcycle who have abstained sexually for at least 3 days, are either instructed to have intercourse or undergo artificial insemination between 6 to 12 hours prior to their routine investigatory laparoscopy. At operation the fluid that normally occupies the Pouch of Douglas is aspirated (Fig. 15.7). An aliquot of this fluid is then treated with twice its volume of 0.01% (w/v) Saponin to lyse the numerous red cells within it. After resuspending the sperm in distilled water, a count is made of the number of sperm present in the washings. An absence of spermatozoa in the flushings correlates well with poor sperm motility and with continuing infertility.

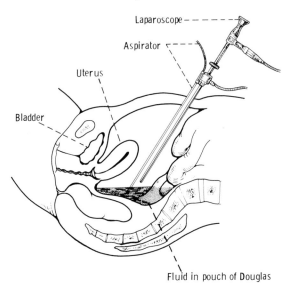

Fig. 15.7. A schematic drawing of the use of the laparoscope to aspirate the fluid from the pouch of Douglas.

Hamster egg penetration test

This is often considered to be the best of all in sperm function tests but it must be remembered that it is very time-consuming and thus very expensive to perform.

In natural circumstances, the fertilization of an oocyte by sperm from another species is prevented by the presence, around the egg, of the zona pellucida. Removal of the zona pellucida may allow penetration of the oocyte by spermatozoa of a totally different species. This is the situation that exists between hamster oocytes and human spermatozoa. The ability of human sperm to penetrate a hamster oocyte from which the zona pellucida has been removed is now being used as a test of the fertilizing ability of human spermatozoa (Yanagamachi *et al.*, 1976). It must be remembered, however, that this test does not accurately mimic human fertilization for it is performed *in vitro* and egg penetration occurs without the sperm having to traverse the zona pellucida. However, from many studies that have now been completed, it is clear that human sperm penetration of zona free hamster oocytes correlates well with the ability of those sperm to penetrate human eggs and produce a pregnancy (Rogers *et al.*, 1979).

Laboratories undertaking this procedure are providing a very valuable service to the clinician. This technique is time-consuming, labour intensive and therefore expensive. Animal house facilities are also necessary. It must be remembered that in Britain at least, *no procedure of any kind* can be performed on any living animal without full licencing and authorization by the Home Office. An outline of the methodology of the 'egg penetration test' is given below:

1. *Preparation of the zona free oocytes*

• To obtain a lot of eggs, the female golden hamster (*Mesocricetus auratus*) must be superovulated with gonadotrophins. On Day 1 of the cycle (manifested by a slight white vaginal discharge) female hamsters are injected intraperitoneally with 25 i.u. of pregnant mares serum gonadotrophin. On Day 3, an intraperitoneal injection of 25 i.u. of human chorionic gonadotrophin (HCG) is given to induce follicular rupture.

• At 17–22 hours (the time seems to depend on the strain of hamster) the animals are killed and their oviducts dissected out. Attached to the ends of the ducts is a mass of oocytes each surrounded by a mass of cumulus cells. After separation from the oviduct this mass of cells is placed in BWW (Bigger, Whitten and Whittingham) medium containing 0.3% human serum albumin.

• The cells are now placed in a BWW medium which contains 0.1% hyaluronidase. This will separate all the cumulus cells leaving the much larger oocytes free in the medium.

• The eggs are now washed twice in BWW and then placed briefly in a 0.1% solution of trypsin in BWW. This will remove the zona pellucida. The eggs are removed and washed in BWW and then placed in BWW under mineral oil in a sterile plastic Petri dish. From each hamster, it is possible using this protocol to obtain between 20–50 eggs from each animal. It is necessary to use 20–30 eggs for each sample of semen tested (Fig. 15.8).

2. *Penetration of the human sperm*

• A fresh semen sample is collected into a sterile jar and incubated for 20 minutes at 37°C until it has liquified. A 5 ml aliquot of BWW is now placed in a sterile capped plastic centrifuge tube. Using a Pasteur pipette around 2 ml of the liquified semen is introduced under the

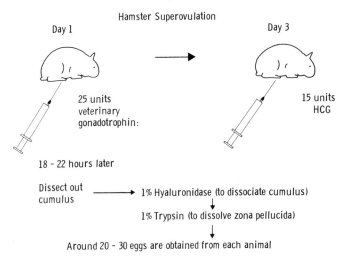

Hamster Superovulation

Day 1

25 units
veterinary
gonadotrophin:

Day 3

15 units
HCG

18 - 22 hours later

Dissect out ———→ 1% Hyaluronidase (to dissociate cumulus)
cumulus   ↓
                    1% Trypsin (to dissolve zona pellucida)
                                    ↓
Around 20 - 30 eggs are obtained from each animal

Fig. 15.8. A diagrammatic representation of the hamster superovulation used in the hamster egg penetration test.

BWW into the bottom of the tube. The semen and the medium thus forms two layers. The tube is now incubated for 1–2 hours at 37°C and this will allow the motile sperm to 'swim up' into the BWW medium thus selecting out sperm of good motility. Throughout the incubation medium is gradually added to the tube to provide a total volume of 10 ml.

• The supernatant is now removed and gently centrifuged at 700 g for 6 minutes and then washed with BWW again. The sperm are now suspended in a volume of medium which will give a concentration of sperm of 10×10^6/ml almost all of which will be motile.

3. In vitro *insemination*

• A volume of 0.2 ml of the sperm suspension is now added, under the mineral oil, to the medium containing the zona free eggs. A sterile technique must be used throughout.
• The eggs and sperm are incubated together for about 12 hours (in the dark at 37°C).

4. *Examination of the eggs*

Using a microscope, the eggs are now aspirated from under the drop of mineral oil to a microscope slide. Apply a coverslip and press down on this moderately hard. The slide is now examined using a microscope and phase contrast optics. If the eggs have been penetrated by sperm, swollen diffuse sperm heads may be seen in the egg which is attached to its accompanying tail (Fig. 15.9). The percentage of the eggs that have been penetrated is then assessed. In semen of good fertility, around 50% of the eggs will have been penetrated.

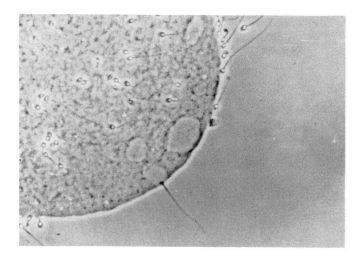

Fig. 15.9. Photomicrograph showing the swollen heads of spermatozoa that have penetrated a zona-free hamster oocyte. The remaining sperm are simply adherent to the surface of the oocyte (by kind permission of Mr J. Pryor, FRCS).

It is possible to fix and strain these eggs and thus provide a permanent record of the test.

'Mixed gamete' assay

As has recently been made clear, there are some spermatozoa which cause failure of conception due to their inability to bind to and penetrate zona pellucida but which have no problem in passing through the membrane into the egg. Such a defect will not manifest itself in the hamster egg penetration test. With this problem in mind, Overstreet *et al.* (1980) devised a 'mixed gamete assay'. In this assay human sperm, zona-free hamster eggs and the zona pellucidae taken from human eggs are incubated together. Such an assay is time-consuming and expensive but may give a realistic appraisal of the fertilizing ability of sperm.

As can be seen from the above, all sperm function tests do need time and attention. However, they are of great value to the clinician and at least the simpler sperm invasion tests should form part of the routine work of a semen analysis laboratory.

References

Alexander, N. (1981) Evaluation of male infertility with an *in-vitro* cervical mucus penetration test. *Fertility and Sterility* **36**, 201–8.

Kremer, J. (1965) A simple sperm penetration test. *International Journal of Fertility* **10**, 209–15.

Kremer, J. & Jager, S. (1976) The Sperm-Cervical Mucus Contact Test: A preliminary report. *Fertility and Sterility* **27**, 335–40.

Odeblad, E. (1968) The functional structure of cervical mucus. *Acta Obstetrica Gynecologica Scandinavica* (Suppl) **47**, 57–9.

Overstreet, J. W., Yanagimachi, R., Katz, D. F., Hayashi, K. & Hanson, F. W. (1980) Penetration of human spermatozoa into human zona pellucida and the zona free hamster egg: A study of fertile donors and infertile patients. *Fertility and Sterility* **33**, 534–42.

Rogers, B. J., Van Campen, H., Ueno, M., Lambert, H., Bronson, R. & Hale, R. (1979) Analysis of human spermatozoa fertilising ability using zona-free ova. *Fertility and Sterility* **32**, 664–70.

Templeton, A. A. & Mortimer, D. (1982) The development of a clinical test of sperm migration to the site of fertilisation. *Fertility and Sterility* **37**, 410–5.

Yanagimachi, R., Yanagimachi, H. & Rogers, B. J. (1976) The use of zona-free animal ova as a test system for the assessment of the fertilising capacity of human spermatozoa. *Biological Reproduction* **15**, 471–6.

16

Cryopreservation of Semen

The cryopreservation of sperm first became a reality when in 1949 Polge and his co-workers discovered that glycerol protected fowl spermatozoa from the otherwise lethal effects of freezing. By applying a variety of different protocols based on the use of glycerol, it then became possible to freeze the sperm of domestic animals and finally to achieve the cryopreservation of human sperm.

Although the cryopreservation of semen does not form part of a routine semen analysis, the ability of a laboratory to freeze semen in liquid nitrogen may considerably enhance the scope of the clinician in the treatment of a couple's infertility. Although cryopreservation is primarily used for the storage of semen for a donor insemination programme, there are also many situations in infertility where the storage of the husband's semen may be valuable in the management of a couple's infertility. Thus although the freezing of sperm within an infertility clinic may not be essential, it is certainly a useful adjunct both to the analysis of semen and to infertility therapy in general. Cryopreservation also has the advantage of being a procedure that is easy to perform and which is rapidly completed. Many laboratories are already able to freeze and store semen and as many other laboratories involved in semen analysis and andrology would like to be able to carry out semen storage if only on a limited scale, a section concerned with cryopreservation of semen is therefore included in this book.

Liquid nitrogen is used for the preservation of sperm for two main reasons.

1 At the temperature of liquid nitrogen ($-196°C$) virtually all metabolic activity completely ceases and thus sperm, at least in theory, can be stored in liquid nitrogen indefinitely.

2 The very low temperature of liquid nitrogen allows for very rapid freezing of the semen sample.

For cryopreservation to be of value, live and functionally competent spermatozoa must be obtained from the semen after thawing. During the course of freezing, the sperm may be killed in two ways. Firstly, each spermatozoon as a cellular module may become damaged by the formation of ice crystals within its nucleus and cytoplasm; as a consequence of ice crystal formation, the cell membranes are disrupted and the sperm is killed. Ice crystal formation may be prevented by a controlled rate of freezing. The sperm may also be damaged during freezing by water loss. During the freezing process, the solidification of water produces an increase in solute concentration both within and also outside the sperm. Thus passage of water in and out of the sperm may occur both during freezing and during thawing which will result in death of the sperm. In order to prevent these osmotic changes, the sperm, prior to freezing, are mixed with a diluent containing glycerol which is highly water soluble and acts as semen cryoprotectant. Glycerol remains in solution as freezing occurs and protects the sperm from these osmotic changes. However, despite these precautions, around one-third of all the motile sperm in a semen specimen will be killed by the freezing process and for this reason poor quality semen will not be improved by freezing.

The need for sperm cryopreservation

There are many reasons why cryopreservation of semen is of value in the management of infertility and some of the possible indications for its use are outlined below.

AID

By far the most common reason for storing sperm in liquid nitrogen is AID. Women undergoing artificial insemination by donor need to be inseminated at mid-cycle. Without using stored semen, the donors would have to produce a semen specimen on days compatible with the patient's ovulation. The logistic and organizational problems this produces are therefore considerable. The cryopreservation of sperm obviates all these problems and is very valuable for use in large insemination programmes.

'Absentee' husbands

A number of husbands now work abroad and may be away from home for many months. In women with fertility problems, treatment, i.e. using expensive drugs, may not be feasible until pregnancy becomes a possibility. In such situations, treatment would have to be delayed until the husband returned home. Storage of the husband's semen for use for insemination at mid-cycle allows the wife's therapy to proceed and even pregnancy to occur in the absence of the consort.

Associated female disorders requiring AIH

In some female patients, particularly those with hostile cervical mucus, artificial insemination using the husband's sperm may be needed to overcome the barrier to the entry of the sperm into the female genital tract. It is indeed best to use fresh semen if possible in this situation but there are some men who find the production of semen specimens each month (and sometimes more than one each month) difficult and distasteful. In these circumstances freezing of their semen helps to avoid the stress and anxiety that the need for semen production 'to order' may induce.

Sexual problems

Problems concerned with sexual intercourse may occur among infertile couples and occasionally the associated infertility may be overcome using semen that has been stored. Thus one specimen can be used to inseminate the female partner over several months without need for the production of further ejaculation.

Neurological disorders

In many patients with neurological disease, ejaculation may be a problem and it may be difficult for the patient to produce a semen specimen. Such semen is thus valuable and, if it can be stored safely, it may be used for insemination in small aliquots for the wife over several cycles. Cryopreservation of such samples of semen may thus enhance the probability of conception very substantially.

Patients about to undergo chemotherapy and radiation treatment

Testicular tumours tend to occur in young men and the surgery and more particularly the subsequent chemotherapy and often radiotherapy will render such men sterile. Storage of semen samples prior to therapy and their use for artificial insemination at a later date will allow patients to complete a family long after the tumour has been successfully treated.

Oligozoospermia

Freezing has also been used in an attempt to concentrate sperm from men with severe oligozoospermia. This procedure however is of little value as sperm from severely oligozoospermic semen rarely survive the freeze (Ledward *et al.*, 1977).

Many other uses for cryopreservation have also been reported, notably the storage of semen prior to vasectomy. It can thus be appreciated that cryopreservation of semen has an important part to play in the management of many aspects of infertility.

Freezing of semen

Many regimes of freezing semen have been described (Trounson *et al.*, 1976). Some involve the use of complex and expensive apparatus while others successfully make use of much simpler equipment and methodology.

Diluents

A number of diluents may be mixed with semen prior to freezing. The diluent may consist of the cryoprotectant, glycerol, alone or it may be made up of a number of different substances.

Glycerol alone 10% vol/vol

Successful cryopreservation may be obtained by using glycerol. The glycerol used must be of the purity laid down by the British Pharmacopoea and industrial glycerol must *not* be substituted. Glycerol is added to produce a 10% solution volume for volume, that is, 9 parts of semen to 1 part of glycerol.

Carlborg–Matheson–Gemzell mixture

This is a more complex diluent but is the one that is used in many AID programmes (Matheson *et al.*, 1969).

The solution is made up of Tri-sodium citrate, glucose, glycerol, egg yolk and glycerine (Table 16.1). The protein in the egg yolk in conjunction with the glycerol is a good cryoprotectant and the citrate and the glucose act as nutrients after thawing. This mixture is added at room temperature to an equal volume of semen, e.g. 5 ml of semen + 5 ml diluent. In some AID programmes an antibiotic (usually Erythromycin) is added in order to avoid any possible transfer of infection from the semen to the recipient.

Table 16.1. The Matheson–Carlborg–Gemzell Medium which is frequently used as a cryoprotectant in many AID programmes

1	Mix together the following solutions:	
	3% Tri-sodium Citrate	39 ml ⎫ dissolved in de-ionized water
	5.5% Glucose	26 ml ⎭
	Glycerol	15 ml
	Fresh egg yolk filtered through gauze	20 ml
2	After thorough mixing, now add	
	Glycine	1.5 g
	Erythromycin	0.1 g
3	Incubate this mixture at 56°C for 30 minutes and then cool to room temperature.	
4	Using a 1.4% solution of sodium bicarbonate, adjust the pH of the mixture to 7.2–7.4.	
5	Store in brown, light-excluding bottles.	

After addition of the diluent to the semen the two must be mixed well. This is best achieved by rolling the semen–diluent mixture in its container or simply by the use of gentle agitation.

It is *very* important to allow the diluent–semen mixture to stand at room temperature for at least 10 minutes in order that the spermatozoa may become well coated by the cryoprotectant.

Semen containers

As the rate of freezing must be evenly distributed, the semen containers must have a small diameter and only hold a small volume of the semen–diluent mixture. Vials may be used into which 0.25–0.5 ml volumes of semen may be stored. Alternatively straws sealed at one end each of which will hold 0.25 ml of the semen–diluent mixture can also be employed. These straws are easy to handle and to store. They are manufactured in nine different colours. The end of each straw is sealed using a polyvinyl alcohol powder which is also available in different colours. Using different coloured straws sealed with different coloured powder provides a large number of colour codes by which one can identify semen and obviate the need for labelling.

The straws are now filled with the semen–diluent mixture using negative pressure. An average specimen of semen when mixed with diluent will fill around 20 straws. The ends of the straws are now sealed by dipping them into the polyvinyl alcohol powder.

Freezing

The rate of freezing is very important. Complex equipment will do this accurately (Fig. 16.1), but similar though less well controlled results may be achieved more simply. A simple method of freezing used by one of the authors (JPC) will now be outlined.

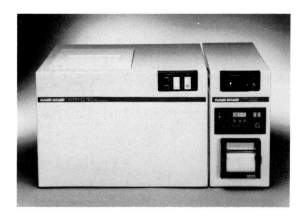

Fig. 16.1. The Planer Kryo 10 controlled rate freezer is an example of an apparatus used for cryopreseration of many types of cells including spermatozoa. This machine can be pre-programmed to freeze at any rate needed. (Reproduced by kind permission of Planer Products Ltd., Sunbury on Thames, Middlesex.)

The first step is to obtain a loss of temperature of 10°C/minute down to a temperature of −70°C. The nitrogen vapour that will lie above liquid nitrogen fortuitously has a temperature of around −70°C. The straws are suspended in liquid nitrogen vapour for 10 minutes which will ensure a temperature drop of around 10°C/minute. At the end of this time they are then plunged into the liquid nitrogen itself.

Storage tanks

The most suitable tanks for use in a small laboratory are those of 34–40 litres in volume (Fig. 16.2). It is *most* important to have narrow necked tanks as this will result in far less nitrogen loss each time the tank is opened. In these tanks, the straws are held in small, divided containers within the liquid nitrogen suspended from the top of the tank (Fig. 16.3). Each 40 litre tank will hold as many as 14 000 (0.25 ml each) straws and thus will be more than adequate for all but the largest AID centres. It is also of value to have smaller storage dewars containing only liquid nitrogen for use as a 'top-up' for the main tank if necessary.

Thawing the straws

Adequate survival is obtained after very rapid thawing. There are several methods described. These include

  1 thawing for 7 seconds at 37°C;

  2 for 15 minutes at room temperature or

  3 placing the semen container under lukewarm tap water for a few seconds. All methods result in approximately the same percentage survival of the sperm.

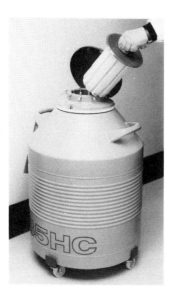

Fig. 16.2. A liquid nitrogen storage tank.

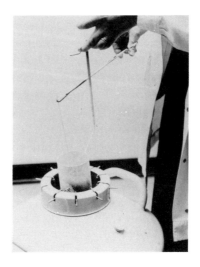

Fig. 16.3. Small containers within the tank which are used to hold individual groups of straws.

Assessing cryosurvival

The percentage survival of sperm in terms of motility is usually reported in relation to the pre-freeze motility. The pre-freeze motility is deemed 100% and the post-thaw motility is reported as a percentage of this pre-freeze motility. Thus if the pre-freeze motility is 60% and the post-thaw motility 30%, the cryosurvival is reported as 50%.

From this short section, it can be seen that even in the absence of an AID service, cryopreservation is of value to the clinician and is simple for an average laboratory to carry out.

References

Ledward, R. S., Crich, J. P., Symonds, E. M. & Cotton, R. E. (1977) The management of oligospermia by freezing and concentration of semen. *IRCS (Med. Sci.)* **5**, 537.

Matheson, G. W., Carlborg, L. & Gemzell, C. (1969) Frozen human semen for artificial insemination. *American Journal of Obstetrics and Gynaecology* **104**, 495–501.

Polge, C., Smith, A. U. & Parkes, A. S. (1949) Revival of spermatozoa after vitrification and dehydration at low temperatures. *Nature* **164**, 666.

Trounson, A. O., Mahadevan, M., Wood, J. & Leeton, J. F. (1976) Studies on the deep freezing and artificial insemination of human semen. In *Frozen Human Semen*, Richardson, D., Joyce, D. & Symonds, E. M. (eds), pp. 173–85. Royal College of Obstetricians and Gynaecologists, London.

17

Computer Assisted Semen Analysis (CASA)

As the preceding chapters in this book should have made clear, the analysis of semen is a complex, time-consuming and technically difficult procedure. Many aspects of semen analysis, in particular those involving both the quantitative and the qualitative evaluation of sperm movement, are based on subjective assessment rather than objective measurement. More objective means of analysing sperm movement can be achieved by the use of photography and by the examination of individual frames of a video micrograph but these methods are extremely tedious and take up much laboratory time.

Semen analysis does however have one advantage: much but not all of the analysis makes use of numbers, and for this reason it should be feasible, and indeed it is possible, to apply computer technology to this problem. If such techniques are applied to semen analysis, more accurate and much more objective means of analysis of semen become available. At the same time it should be possible to carry out most of a semen analysis in much greater detail in a very short time.

In the past, systems linking a computer to a semen analysis have been devised. Still photographs of sperm have been projected onto a digitizer and the number of sperm, together with their mean size and their different shapes could then be calculated by a computer. This system had the disadvantage that still photography was again required, limiting its application in a busy pathology laboratory. Moreover, this method was not easily applicable to the analysis of sperm movement.

More recently, the same type of analysis could be performed by examining individual frames of a video-micrograph either directly or after their projection onto a digitizer pad. It is also possible to examine still photographs on video frames using a light pen on a light sensitive screen. However, although these methods provide much more objective methods of examining spermatozoa and their movement, they are only marginally less time-consuming than those

143

techniques involving direct measurements of video or photographic images.

The computer analysis of reflected laser light from spermatozoa has also been described (Jouannet *et al.*, 1977). The analysis of the number of reflections of the laser light from the sperm allow an estimate of their numbers and to some extent their size. From the analysis of repeated pulses of laser light, it is possible for the computer to calculate the number of moving sperm within a sample, their linearity and also their velocity. This excellent but costly system produces an extremely rapid analysis of sperm movement, but has the disadvantage that it can provide little information concerning sperm morphology.

The most recent development in the application of computer technology to semen analysis involves video image motion analysis. This seems to be the most promising of all the new techniques and will be described in more detail below.

Video Image Motion Analysis

In these systems, the best of which is *CellSoft*, devised by Cryo Resources Ltd., New York, USA, the computer analyses a semen sample over a short period of time usually utilizing around 15 frames of videotape or a time interval of 0.75 seconds. In this way the system can analyse many aspects of sperm movement very rapidly indeed. Computer assisted examination of several fields allows the examination of large numbers of sperm in a very short time. An analysis of each field is generated in under 1 minute. Software is also available to analyse the lateral head displacement that is seen during sperm movement and this may be important in the overall assessment of the potential fertility of a semen sample (Aitken *et al.*, 1985). Using this system, it is also possible to analyse sperm size and shape and thus provide a very rapid and objective analysis of sperm morphology.

The apparatus

The semen can be analysed either directly or by means of pre-recorded video-micrography. The system therefore has the advantage that, provided a video-micrograph is taken of the semen on its arrival at the laboratory, the actual computer assisted semen analysis can be carried out long after the semen was delivered to the hospital. It also has the advantage that if such a video-micrograph is kept in store, it is possible to 're-examine' a sample at a later date if so required. This feature may be of particular value in a research programme.

Counting chamber

An aliquot of the well mixed sample of semen to be examined is placed in a chamber of exactly 10 μm deep in order to ensure that sperm movement remains unimpeded, and to allow the computer to calculate the number of sperm present per unit volume of seminal fluid. For this purpose a Makler or a CellSoft Chamber must be employed.

Stage warmer

As this system will analyse sperm velocity, and as sperm velocity is much affected by temperature, a warmer for the microscope stage is needed to ensure that the semen is examined at a known temperature. A stage warmer set to provide a temperature of 37 or 38°C is commonly employed. The semen sample must also be allowed time to reach this temperature prior to the analysis.

Microscope

A standard laboratory microscope, provided it has a photographic port, can be used. Phase contrast optics are also necessary.

Videocamera and video cassette recorder

A black and white videocamera is fitted to the photographic port of the microscope. The images so obtained may pass directly to the computer or into a standard video cassette recorder. A commonly used format is best employed as this will allow you to analyse video cassette tapes that may be sent to your laboratory from other centres.

Television monitors

Two black and white television monitors are used in this system, one to provide the actual images of the semen sample, and the other to provide the digitally converted image derived from the computer itself.

The hardware

The hardware for which the software in these systems has been designed are simple microcomputers. However, larger systems may also be used. Interfaced with this computer is a picture store and a hard disc. Further memory may be added in order to store all the data derived from this system if this is desired.

The printer

The results of the analysis are displayed on the computer screen or can be printed out on any standard computer printer. The movement, shape and size of each individual sperm analysed can also be obtained on a print out.

This whole system is depicted in Fig. 17.1.

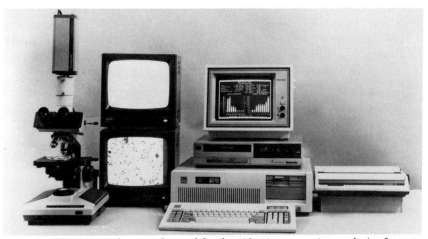

Fig. 17.1. The system that may be used for the video image motion analysis of semen (Published by kind permission of Cryo Resources, Ltd., 701 Seventh Avenue, New York, USA.)

The software

The software designed by Cryo Resources, New York, USA, is available in a series of packages. Individual packages examine sperm number, aspects of sperm movement and sperm morphology. By altering the parameters at which the computer is set, it is possible to apply this software to the semen of other mammals with similarly shaped spermatozoa, e.g. bull, stallion, boar or ram. Software packages are now also available for the examination of rodent semen and this may be of value to those involved in a wide variety of toxicological studies.

The analysis

The software provides an analysis of the number of spermatozoa per millilitre, the number of motile and non-motile sperm and the percentage of motile sperm (Fig. 17.2). It also calculates the mean velocity and draws a distribution histogram of the speed of individual spermatozoa in microns per second (Fig. 17.3). The mean straight line velocity is calculated and from these figures the mean linearity is calculated. The linearity is an empirical assessment of the 'straightness' of the progress of sperm and thus is a function of that commonly known as progressive activity. A distribution histogram of the linearity of individual spermatozoa is also drawn (Fig. 17.3). Software is also available which examines the lateral head displacement and beat/cross frequency.

Using pre-set parameters, some software can also analyse the size and shape of sperm heads and thus provide an analysis of sperm morphology which can also be presented graphically as distribution histograms of each of the individual cell types.

Although these systems are at present installed only in a small number of centres, they represent a major advance in the analysis of semen. Not only are they capable of completing an assessment of many of the variables, such as sperm velocity, much more rapidly than would be possible photographically but they also provide, at long last, an objective method of examining seminal fluid. Systems such as these will one day certainly replace many of the 'guesstimates' in semen analysis and are likely to provide us with a better differentiation between fertile and infertile semen.

```
# Cells Analysed  : 235       (cells)    Mean Velocity    : 46.820  (microns/sec)
Concentration     : 81.704    (mill/ml)   SD,      SEM    : 24.772      2.671
# Mot.,# Non-Mot.: 170,65     (cells)    Mean Linearity   : 5.312
Percent Motility  : 72.34     (%)         SD,      SEM    : 3.215       0.346
Conc. Motile      : 59.105    (mill/ml)  Mot. Index       : 33.870  (microns/sec)
```

Fig. 17.2. A print out of an individual semen analysis (reproduced by kind permission of Leycor Laboratories, 11 Regent Street, Nottingham)

Chapter 17

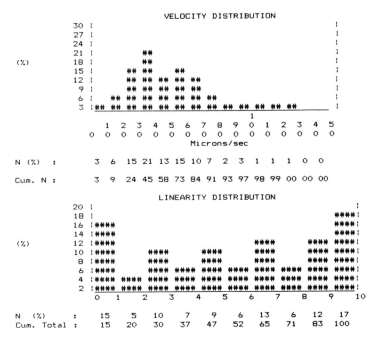

Fig. 17.3. A distribution histogram of (a) the velocities (μm/second) of individual spermatozoa and (b) the linearities of individual spermatozoa. (Reproduced by kind permission of Leycor Laboratories, 11 Regent Street, Nottingham)

Accessing computer systems that analyse semen

Computer systems that analyse seminal fluid are at present expensive but it must be remembered that they can, for a small investment, be made available for use by smaller laboratories with restricted finance. A number of possible methods of accessing these systems are described below:

Videotape

If a black and white video camera and a video taperecorder (preferably of industrial quality) are purchased, video-micrographic tape recordings of seminal fluid can be made and the tape sent by post for analysis to a centre where such a system is available. In this way not only will there be an improvement in the semen analysis but a great saving of time and effort will be made in many pathology laboratories on time-consuming and difficult cell counts and cell analyses.

Television transmission

A much more rapid, but much more costly approach would be to beam a television picture of the semen to the central laboratory. This technique would allow an immediate analysis to be performed. The cost of this system at present is prohibitive but such means of accessing central computers must be under consideration in the future.

Telephone modems

At present it is possible, using a modem, to transmit still pictures down a telephone line. The analysis of semen, however, requires the transmission of moving pictures and to date no modem of sufficient power and speed is available to transmit video frames at the speed needed to carry out this type of analysis. Nevertheless, great improvements are being made in the power of modems, and it is likely that such a method of delivering information to computers as well as accessing them will be available in the future.

Computer assisted semen analysis is an exciting new pathological examination which has an important future. It will be time saving in a routine laboratory and will play a vital role in many research projects involving the evaluation of mammalian seminal fluid. It will also provide a method of semen analysis which would be available to otherwise untrained laboratory personnel.

References

Aitken, R. J., Sutton, M., Warner, P. & Richardson, D. W. (1985). Relationship between the movement characteristics of human spermatozoa and their ability to penetrate cervical mucus and zona-free oocytes. *Journal of Reproduction and Fertility* **73,** 441–9.

Jouannet, P., Valochine, B., Dequent, P., Semes, C. & David, E. (1977) Light scattering determination of various characteristic parameters of spermatozoa motility in a series of human sperm. *Andrologia* **9** 36–49.

Index